W0037729

Rules and Tools for Parents of Children With Autism Spectrum and Related Disorders: Changing Behavior One Step at a Time

Trillium Creek Primary School
1025 SW Rosemont Road
West Linn, OR 97068

Judith Coucouvanis, MA, NP, PMHCNS-BC

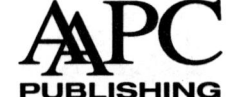

PUBLISHING

P.O. Box 23173
Shawnee Mission, Kansas 66283-0173
www.aapcpublishing.net

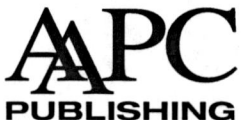

©2015 AAPC Publishing
P.O. Box 23173
Shawnee Mission, Kansas 66283-0173
www.aapcpublishing.net

All rights reserved. No part of the material protected by this copyright notice may be reproduced or used in any form or by any means, electronic or mechanical, including photocopying, recording, or by any information storage and retrieval system, without the prior written permission of the copyright owner.

Publisher's Cataloging-in-Publication

Coucouvanis, Judith.

   Rules and tools for parents of children with autism spectrum and related disorders : changing behavior one step at a time / Judith Coucouvanis. -- Shawnee Mission, Kansas : AAPC Publishing, [2014]

       pages ; cm.
       ISBN: 978-1-937473-85-3
       LCCN: 2014948827
       Includes bibliographical references and index.
       Summary: This book gives parents the tools they need to develop their child's behavior intervention and skill development plans. A major focus is on helping parents answer the question: What can I do that will help my child be successful? Topics include behavior, communication, reward systems, social skills, and medication support.--Publisher.

       1. Parents of autistic children--Handbooks, manuals, etc. 2. Autism spectrum disorders in children--Treatment. 3. Asperger's syndrome in children--Treatment. 4. Autism in children--Treatment. 5. Sensory integration dysfunction in children--Treatment. 6. Autistic children-- Education. 7. Asperger's syndrome--Patients--Education. 8. Children with autism spectrum disorders--Education. 9. Social skills in children-- Study and teaching. 10. Language disorders in children--Treatment. I. Title.

RJ506.A9 C687 2014
918.92/858832--dc23   1409

Visual Support art: LessonPix; www.lessonpix.com

Characters: ©NVTech; www.nvtech.com

Black and white art and Photographs: ©Thinkstock Photos; www.thinkstockphotos.com

This book is designed in Myriad Pro.

Printed in the United States of America.

Acknowledgments

I am deeply grateful to the many persons with autism, parents, grandparents, caretakers of children with autism, and colleagues who are the inspiration for this book, and the many families who contributed by sharing their personal rules and tools. In addition, I am especially appreciative to my dear friend Dorothy Peacor, colleagues Greg Hanna and Michelle Keyes, and my daughters, Electra Coucouvanis and Kathryn Alba, who took time from their very busy schedules to provide extremely valuable comments. Their unique perspectives strengthened the book, making it easier to read and even more practical. I thank them for their collective and invaluable wisdom.

Foreword

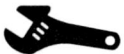

More than 50% of children and adolescents with autism spectrum disorder (ASD) experience challenges in regulating their behavior, resulting in "behavior" problems (Farmer et al., 2014; Mazurek, Kanne, & Wodka, 2013). The right interventions provide positive learning opportunities and happier, well-regulated children. The wrong interventions provide stress for families and their children and negatively impact self-esteem, social interactions, leisure skills, academic performance, and ultimately the ability to have a high quality of life.

This book is about the right interventions.

If parents of children with ASD can buy only one book, this should be the one. It is right on target. Coucouvanis' comprehensive understanding of ASD, her joy and skill in supporting families and learners on the spectrum, and her respect for families are clearly communicated in this easy-to-use book. She offers a realistic and positive way of viewing "behavior" and tools to help individuals on the autism spectrum reach their potential.

Coucouvanis also demystifies the terminology and procedures used by education and mental health systems. Family members who read this book will have the tools to better understand their child's challenges and strengths, be able to participate more actively in individualized education program (IEP) meetings, and understand the best practices in education.

Parent-implemented interventions have been identified as an evidence-based practice by National Autism Center (NAC, 2009), National Professional Development Center on ASD (NPDC on ASD, n.d.), and Centers for Medicare and Medicaid Services (CMS, 2010). To date, few resources have seriously viewed parents as change agents for their children by providing easy-to-use yet comprehensive tools. This book gives parents the much-needed information that will empower them to be their child's best advocates and will ultimately lead to their child reaching his or her limitless potential.

> – **Brenda Smith Myles, PhD,** consultant with the Ohio Center for Autism and Low Incidence (OCALI) and Ziggurat Group; author and international speaker.

References

Centers for Medicare and Medicaid Services. (2010). *Autism spectrum disorders: Final report on environmental scan.* Washington, DC: Author.

Farmer, C., Butter, E., Mazurek, M. O., Cowan, C., Lainhart, J., Cook, E. H., DeWitt, M. B., & Aman, M. (2014). Aggression in children with autism spectrum disorders and a clinic-referred group. *Autism.* doi: 10.1177/1362361313518995

Mazurek, M. O., Kanne, S. M., & Wodka, E. L. (2013). Physical aggression in children and adolescents with autism spectrum disorders. *Research in Autism Spectrum Disorders, 7*(3), 455-465.

National Autism Center. (2009). *National standards report: Addressing the need for evidence-based practice guidelines for autism spectrum disorders.* Randolph, MA: Author.

National Professional Development Center on Autism Spectrum Disorders. (n.d.). *Evidence-based practice briefs.* Retrieved from http://autismpdc.fpg.unc.edu/content/briefs

TABLE OF CONTENTS

Introduction..1

Chapter 1: Behavior and Autism 11

Chapter 2: The Problem 15

Chapter 3: Is the Behavior Significant? 25

Chapter 4: Determining Why: Reasons for the Behavior................................ 39

Chapter 5: The Power of Antecedents 53

Chapter 6: Effective Communication 65

Chapter 7: Teaching New Rules 81

Chapter 8: Using Praise and Primary Rewards 93

Chapter 9: Using Secondary Rewards 109

Chapter 10: Building Flexibility 119

Chapter 11: Changing Routines and Fixations 133

Chapter 12: "Now and Forever".. 141

Chapter 13: Teaching Social Skills: Part I – Introduction................................ 163

Chapter 14: Teaching Social Skills: Part II – The Tools.................................. 177

Chapter 15: Using Consequences 195

Chapter 16: Medication Support 209

Chapter 17: The Final Chapter: Putting It All Together................................... 223

Appendix I: Complete List of the Rules... 237

Appendix II: Relating the Tools to the NAC Standards Report......................... 243

Appendix III: Helpful Information 249

Index.. 257

Introduction

My initiation to the world of autism began 35 years ago in a child and adolescent psychiatric inpatient unit at a university. While there, I had the opportunity to work with many experts (including professionals, care takers, and children), who introduced me to the importance of intensive behavior intervention and skill teaching. I left knowing that children with autism can learn, as long as we know how to teach them.

Since then, I have continued working with families of children with autism, developmental disabilities, and a variety of mental health concerns. I have learned more about autism, including the interaction with other conditions, such as autism and anxiety, but my primary focus has remained on intervention, including social skills training, toilet learning, medication management, and teaching independent skills, as well as behavioral interventions and supports. Eventually, my cumulative knowledge and experience in two very specific areas – social skills training and toilet learning – grew into two books: *Super Skills: A Social Skills Group Program for Children With Asperger Syndrome, High-Functioning Autism and Related Challenges* (2005) and *The Potty Journey: Guide to Toilet Training Children with Special Needs, Including Autism and Related Disorders* (2008).

Many people encouraged me to write this book about behavioral interventions for parents of children with autism, in part because, unfortunately, not everyone has regular access to knowledgeable and experienced treatment providers. My inspiration for the book comes from the countless families who shared, and those who continue to share, their life journeys with me. Most of their names have been changed, yet their stories are an integrated part of this book.

In the last 20 years, the number of children diagnosed with autism has steadily increased. In 2014, the Centers for Disease control reported that 1 in 68 children has been identified. Autism is reported to occur in all racial, ethnic and socioeconomic groups. (http://www.cdc.gov/ncbddd/autism/data.html). With steadily growing numbers, and an increasing demand for services, a wealth of information has emerged about autism and interventions. Yet, according to the National Institute of Mental Health, there is "no single best treatment for all children with ASD (http:// www.nimh.nih.gov/health/topics/autism-spectrum-disorders-pervasive-developmental-disorders/index. shtml). Each child requires individualized, systematic, and comprehensive treatment.

In 2009, the National Autism Center (NAC) published a thorough investigation of current research and practices in the fields of educational and behavioral treatment for persons with autism under age 22. One purpose was to provide the most up-to-date information to those who must make complex decisions when selecting autism treatment(s). The committee created a four-tier rating system to describe the level of effectiveness of a total of 38 autism treatments. The full report is available at http://www.nationalautismcenter.org/pdf/NAC%20Standards%20Report.pdf.

Several treatments were found to have favorable outcomes towards increasing skills and reducing problem behavior, the primary focus of *Rules and Tools for Parenting Children With Autism Spectrum and Related Disorders*. While the tools in this book have not undergone rigorous research, they are derived from research-based principles and can be related to both Established and Emerging Treatments in the NAC report. The relationship(s) of each rule to its main corresponding NAC treatment category is described in Appendix II.

About This Book

As a parent of a child with autism, you face a daunting array of choices and decisions, maybe without consistent professional guidance. Perhaps your child is on a waiting list for services, and you are having to wait weeks or even months for an appointment, leaving you feeling stressed and worried about your child's future. Perhaps you are overwhelmed trying to determine which interventions and treatments are best for your child. Whom should you trust? What will give you hope?

In an ideal world, you would have an expert to guide you; however, in many communities there is a shortage of qualified professionals. This book is written to give you the tools you need to begin to develop your child's behavior intervention and skill development plans. In other words, to enable you to answer the question: What can I try that might help my child be successful? My goal is that you learn to think differently about your child's behavior. If what you are doing isn't working, then this book is for you. Step by step, this book gives you tools that will help you think about and explore your child's behaviors from a fresh perspective. In particular, you are encouraged to begin to notice and examine the multitude of variables that influence behavior so you can increase your ability to prevent problems in the first place. The goal here is to help you to feel empowered by introducing you to the process of behavior change so that when you have access to professional guidance you have a better understanding of the language of behavior in general, and your child's behavior in particular.

Before you can start to expect successful behavior change in your child, you need to perfect your own detective skills. This book will show you how to observe for behaviors and gather information so that you can collaborate with others to find effective solutions to problems. You will likely also have to modify your own behavior. You will learn to focus more on your parenting and the things you can do differently to solve problems and help your child learn new skills, and less on what is "wrong" with your child. You need new tools for your Parenting Toolkit and new rules to guide your journey.

In this book you will learn:

1. Why you must think about the future (Chapter 1)

2. How to identify a specific problem and determine its significance (Chapters 1-3)

3. Why you must figure out the reason(s) for a problem (Chapters 1 & 4)

4. How to adjust your expectations to fit your child (Chapter 4)

5. How to set up the environment to prevent problems in the first place (Chapters 5 & 6)

6. Effective communication tools (Chapter 6)

7. The significance of new rules and routines (Chapters 7 & 11)

8. How to build flexibility with preparation (Chapter 10)

9. How to change routines and fixations (Chapter 11)

10. The significance of "now and forever" routines and how to develop them (Chapter 12)

11. What to do instead of scolding and what to use instead of negative consequences (Chapters 8, 9, & 15)

12. The importance of social skills training (Chapters 13 & 14)

13. The purpose and use of medications (Chapter 16)

14. How to use the 42 tools (Chapters 1-17)

Step by step, *Rules and Tools* will help guide your journey toward greater understanding of your child's behavior. You will need to modify the tools to fit your own situation and your child's circumstances. Ideally, you have the help of a highly qualified professional to guide you through the process. The Helpful Information at the end of the book offers some suggestions of where to look for such guidance. Each child with autism is unique, and behaviors are usually very complex. Yet, your child CAN learn, and with these 118 rules and tools in your Parenting Toolkit, you will be able begin to help him or her.

While reading *Rules and Tools,* you will encounter multiple case examples of real children and their individual situations, although the names, ages, and other details may have been changed. Occasionally, I mention my role in a given situation. In some chapters, you will also read testimonials from families who share their personal rules and tools. Finally, at the end of each chapter you will have an opportunity to develop your own Action Plan by identifying the specific Rules and Tools from that chapter you will try. At the end of the book, you will develop your child's personal MAP: Master Action Plan.

Let's get started!

Chapter 1:
Behavior and Autism

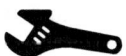

We all have unique personalities guided by our individual temperaments and distinct developmental characteristics. Many of us are extremely energetic, distractible, or impulsive. Others are quiet and withdrawn. Some of us are funny, while others are not. All of us are occasionally angry or upset. Some people have oral language while others have none. A few have diverse and extraordinary cognitive, sensory, and physical abilities or constraints. Some of us have severe fears and anxiety, while others have no fear whatsoever. Whatever the particular collection of attributes may be, these distinct and diverse features influence our behavior.

What Is Behavior Anyway?

Behaviors are actions; something that someone does. The simplest way to identify a behavior is by looking at what we see. An individual who is withdrawn or anxious might spend a great deal of time alone reading or listening to music. Someone who is angry might slam doors, hit, or scream. A person who has no language might protest by hitting his head with his hand. One who is depressed might give away personal possessions. Somebody who is afraid might not sleep at night.

✿ RULE: Behavior communicates.

Behavior is one way of communicating your thoughts and feelings; for example, when you smile, those around you can see that you are happy. When you cry, they see (and hear) that you are sad or upset. Smiling and other "nonverbal" behaviors, such as frowning, pacing, or pointing, communicate just as successfully as verbal behaviors, such as growling, yelling, crying, or talking.

For some people, like many with autism, behavior is the only way they have to communicate. Have you ever been to a foreign country? One where you did not speak the language? If you have, you probably experienced what it feels like to struggle to make someone understand you when you want or need something, like a drink of water or directions to a pharmacy or a bathroom. In a very small way, your experience mirrors a child with autism who is trying to communicate.

Behaviors (and sometimes the individual who displays them) are at times described with adjectives such as "good" or "bad," "positive" or "negative," "appropriate" or "inappropriate," "adaptive" or "maladaptive," "social" or "antisocial," "friendly" or "unfriendly," and so on, depending upon one's point of view.

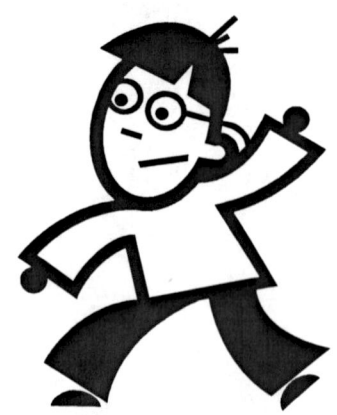

Generally, "good" (or positive) behaviors are actions like saying hello, sharing, helping out, compromising, taking turns, and playing fair, whereas "bad" (or negative) behaviors are actions like hurting oneself or others, lying, cheating, taking things without permission, or teasing to hurt somebody's feelings. Bad behaviors also include behaviors that are socially inappropriate, such as touching your genitals in public places, drooling, or eating non-food items. Behaviors evoke responses from other people; positive behaviors are usually received with positive reactions whereas negative behaviors evoke negative reactions. Some negative behaviors, such as stealing or attacking someone, can become significant "problem behaviors" and even be against the law.

⚙ RULE: Most children learn behaviors from their environment.

Most children learn behaviors and behavioral responses from their environment. Children do not know what is acceptable and unacceptable when they are born. They watch how we behave and how we treat them and other people. As parents, we set up rules and expectations, such as "first finish your homework, then you can watch TV" or "first eat your dinner, then you can have dessert." We offer choices and praise our children for complying with what we ask them to do.

When we are consistent in our behavior and follow through with consequences, most of our children learn to "behave" – follow directions and trust that we will follow through. They learn to feel good about themselves and the world they live in. For typically developing children, when we are reasonably consistent in our expectations, these approaches work.

By the time children are 7 or 8 years old, most are expected to exhibit positive behavior for the majority of the day. By the time they are 12 or 13 years old, children are often held legally accountable for their actions. They are expected to follow the standard rules of human conduct and live respectfully with others in society. When they reach 18 years of age, children become adults, and most receive all of the privileges and rights that adults obtain. They also assume equal responsibilities.

Youth with autism are just like other children when they are born; they do not automatically know acceptable and unacceptable behaviors. These have to be taught, and it is everyone's job to do the teaching. For parents, this is part of parenting. For teachers, this is part of the daily curriculum. Opportunities to learn and practice appropriate behavior are available everywhere.

Setting up the environment so that your child can be successful is a powerful teaching tool and one you will learn about in this book. All of us want our children to become independently functioning adults. However, each child with autism follows a different developmental path – one that is unique and uncharted and contains distinct challenges and different expectations, both for you as parent and your child.

Children With Autism

Evelyn, age 9, is very anxious about her schoolwork. At night she repeats over and over, "I'm a failure." She is distressed any time one of her papers has corrections on it, and it is becoming harder and harder for her parents to convince her to do her homework.

Jack, age 6, asks his mother for some ice cream after dinner for dessert. She gives him the ice cream, and he immediately stamps his feet, growls, and stomps about the house.

Three-year old Abal wears a hijab, a traditional Arabic headscarf. Even though it is not required at her young age, she fights anyone who tries to remove it from her head. Abal has an infant brother, and her parents are very concerned because she pushes and tries to hit him.

⚙ **RULE: No two children with autism are alike.**

Autism is a behavioral diagnosis. This means a child shares this diagnosis with other children because of specific behavioral criteria, including impaired social interactions, impaired verbal and nonverbal communication, and repetitive behaviors. This does not mean that one child will act or behave in the same exact way as other children with autism, as Evelyn, Jack, and Abal illustrate. In fact, no two children with autism are alike; all have varying degrees of functioning along the autism "spectrum." At present, there are no blood tests to confirm the diagnosis. Diagnosis is based upon observing a child's behavior and by interviewing those who know the child.

⚙ **RULE: Children with autism share a unique set of behavior characteristics, yet there are no "typical" behavior challenges.**

Children with autism are different from each other and from other children. Each perceives the world in his or her special way and reacts accordingly. Children with autism don't respond to the environment in the same predictable fashion as typically developing children. Their responses may seem unpredictable and unusual, sometimes bizarre, and frequently successful, even if undesirable. This uniqueness is what makes each child with autism so special; it is also what makes parenting so challenging and solving problems so complicated.

⚙ **RULE: Interventions that work for one child with autism may not work for another.**

Each child's behavior challenges are complex, typically related to many factors and usually well established. They are not random, but purposeful and meaningful. Therefore, interventions that help one child with autism may not help another. Each intervention needs to be tailored to fit the child's unique profile of characteristics. Some strategies are "good fits;" others are not.

Learning to understand your child's unique features and responses is critical if you are going to help him or her develop appropriate skills and behavior. Don't compare your child with autism to other children with autism. Your child has his or her own personal needs. Discover your child's profile of individual and distinct strengths and weaknesses and don't worry about how he or she compares to others.

Gaining Perspective

Parents of children with autism who exhibit problem behavior often ask me, "Won't he grow out of it?" The hope is that with the passage of time, the child's behaviors will become more appropriate or even disappear. The answer is usually a resounding "No!" Most children with autism like predictability and routine. Therefore, once a behavior pattern becomes established, it is often difficult to change, because it is a predictable routine for the child.

⚙ RULE: Children with autism like predictability and routine.

It doesn't matter how wrong, bizarre, age inappropriate, or uncomfortable you think the behavior routine is, the child will continue it indefinitely unless he decides to change it, and that might never happen. This is why some children with autism are called rigid or inflexible. If left alone, their behavior routines become set in cement. (And you know how hard that is to break!)

> *Maria is 5 years old. She has her bowel movements in a diaper while holding on to her mother's hand on top of the cat tree behind the front door of their house. Maria refuses to use the toilet. Her mother is afraid to insist because Maria can become very aggressive when pushed to do something she doesn't want to do. She also has a history of constipation and withholding bowel movements, which adds to her mother's fears.*

> *Tommy has watched* Sesame Street *after school on television since he was 2 years old. He is now 15. He had a tantrum whenever anyone changed the channel, so his parents bought him a television set for his bedroom. Now he doesn't want to come out of his room, and he doesn't want to watch anything else.*

The second reason why children usually don't "grow out" of problem behavior is also related to their rigid routines. Some children with autism are "rule bound." This means that they follow the rules, right? Not always. In my experience, when children with autism do not know or understand the rules, they make up their own. Experts speculate that imposing their personal structure or rules helps children to cope with a world they don't understand, or perhaps the routine is simply a pattern that has become a habit and it is difficult for the person to break it, despite pressure from others to change.

> *Owen insists that his older brothers leave the kitchen table every night after dinner. The lights in the kitchen must be turned off. If they try to stay in the kitchen to do their homework or other activity, Owen becomes angry.*

> *Jordan's parents try everything they can think of to get him to try new foods. He refuses. His rule is that he can only eat white foods.*

To others, Owen and Jordan's behavior seems irrational or illogical. But to them, the rules are making life predictable, and *their rules apply every time the same situation occurs*. It is common for a child's routines to convert into rules and his rules to convert into routines, making behavior change a serious challenge.

For some children, their personal rules and routines govern their actions – not the rules that parents or teachers have set. These frequently irrational rules may become set in stone and, therefore, are very difficult to manage. This excessive resistance to change is one of the diagnostic features of autism. We talk more about, inflexibility, rigidity, and rules in future chapters.

Executive Function

One theory that explains the difficulty that children with autism have with flexibility is executive dysfunction. "Executive function" is a broad term that describes a group of important mental tasks that are regulated by multiple brain structures, including the prefrontal regions of the frontal lobes of the brain. Executive function allows us to make plans, keep track of time, stay on task, shift from task to task, evaluate ideas, solve problems, change our minds, or ask for help. When problems in these areas become so extreme that they interfere with everyday functioning, the person is said to experience a problem with executive functioning, which implies the need for intervention.

Rule of Five

I attended a conference a few years ago that focused on how to support adolescents and adults with autism as they move out of their homes into the community. The speaker described behavior challenges and rigid routines in his adult clients similar to those I see in children and teens, such as restricted eating, self-injurious behavior, tantrums, and aggression. The difference is, of course, that the adults are bigger and can hurt someone or themselves. My personal take-home message was: We have to work smarter to reduce/modify or eliminate behavior challenges in children, because otherwise those problems will still be there 10 or 20 years later.

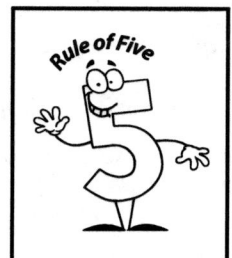

"Oh, she has been doing it forever." This is the answer I often get from parents when I ask how long their child has engaged in a certain behavior. My next question typically is, "Will it be O.K. if she is still doing this in five years?"

Rule of Five

When considering how important a behavior is today, ask yourself whether or not it will be a problem if it continues to occur five years from now. If it will definitely be a problem in five years, mark it as a behavior to change.

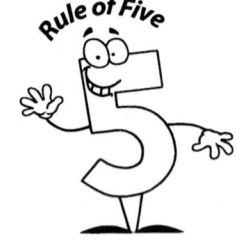

In addition, when you plan to teach your child a new skill or behavior, look to the future and make sure that everything you plan to teach will apply and be appropriate as your child ages. First think about 5 years from now, and then 10 years from now.

⚙ RULE: The Rule of Five: Predict five weeks, five months, and five years into the future.

The Rule of Five helps focus on the bigger picture – How likely is it that the behavior/routine/rule will help or interfere with your child's future skill development? To become independently functioning adults, youth with autism must learn an endless list of skills, so focus on what will be useful in the long term. Everything you do can make a difference. Where do you want your child to be five years from now? What skills does your child need to learn? What can you accomplish today that will help him tomorrow? How can you set your child up to be successful?

This Rule of Five may seem overwhelming, especially when you are struggling just to get through today. However, you can save precious time in the long run when the solution you decide upon, and therefore your child's new behavior, remains appropriate in five years.

☑ To Do: Determine the Rule of Five

Take any one of your child's current behaviors and apply the Rule of Five; ask yourself the following questions:

☐ If this behavior continues, will it be a problem in five weeks, in five months, in five years?

☐ Will this behavior/routine/rule help or hinder future (educational, vocational, personal) opportunities for my child?

Sometimes behaviors that we think are problems now won't be problems in the future, when our child is an adult. One example that comes to mind is greeting. Occasionally, early-elementary children imitate adults and offer to shake hands in greeting. I usually don't insist that parents spend a lot of time and energy trying to teach more age-appropriate greetings. After all, when the child is a teenager, shaking hands will be appropriate. There are so many skills to work on that our time and energy are best spent on those that truly matter as the child ages.

I was in a kindergarten classroom many years ago at Thanksgiving time. The girls were given pictures of girl pilgrims to color and the boys were given pictures of boy pilgrims. The little girl I was observing wanted a boy pilgrim, and when the teacher insisted she color a girl pilgrim, she had a meltdown. In my opinion, this was a Rule of Five moment. It would not have mattered in five days, five weeks, or five months whether or not the girl had colored a girl or a boy pilgrim, and it certainly wouldn't have mattered in five years. Sometimes we adults are just as, or even more, rigid than the children with autism. Choose your battles wisely and engage in those that matter!

We will talk more about rules and routines and the Rule of Five in subsequent chapters, but let's introduce the steps to changing your child's behavior. These are detailed for you in Illustration 1:1. You may wish to copy and laminate the steps so that you can easily refer to them. Each step and the tools you need to implement it are the subject of subsequent chapters in this book.

Illustration 1:1
Steps to Successful Behavior Change

1. Gather information:
   a. What is the problem?
   b. How severe is the problem?
   c. What might be possible reason(s) for the problem?
   d. What might be antecedents to the problem?
   e. What might be underlying variables that contribute to the problem?

2. Focus on prevention:
   a. How could I modify the antecedents?
   b. How could I modify my communication?

3. Focus on change:
   a. What are the replacement behavior(s) and new rule(s) needed right now?
   b. What praise and reinforcement system will I use?
   c. How can I alter routines and fixations?
   d. How can I build flexibility?
   e. What are the negative consequences, if any?

4. Focus on teaching:
   a. What Now and Forever Skills and routines will I teach today?
   b. What appropriate social behavior and skills will I teach today?

5. Will I consider medication supports?

6. How will I evaluate the plan's effectiveness?

⚙ **Action Plan for Chapter 1: Behavior and Autism**
(Select From the Choices Below)

⚙ **Rules to Remember:**

☐ **Behavior communicates.**

☐ **Most children learn behaviors from their environment.**

☐ **No two children with autism are alike.**

☐ **Children with autism share a unique set of behavior characteristics, yet there are no "typical" behavior challenges.**

☐ **Interventions that work for one child with autism may not work for another.**

☐ **Children with autism like predictability and routine.**

☐ **The Rule of Five: Predict five weeks, five months, and five years into the future.**

⚙ **To Do:**

Think of a problem behavior and apply the Rule of Five. Will it matter in five weeks, five months, or five years? Why or why not?

_____

Let's move on to Chapter 2 and the first step of your journey – how to describe the problem.

References and Further Reading

American Psychiatric Association. (2013). *Diagnostic and statistical manual of mental disorders, fifth edition.* Washington, DC: Author.

Aspy, R., & Grossman, B. G. (2012). *Designing comprehensive interventions for high-functioning individuals with autism spectrum disorders: The Ziggurat model. Textbook edition.* Shawnee Mission, KS: AAPC Publishing.

Coucouvanis, J., Hallas, D., Farley, J. (2012). Autism spectrum disorder. In E. L. Yearwood, G. S. Pearson, & J. A. Newland (Eds.), *Child and adolescent behavioral health: A resource for advanced practice psychiatric and primary care practitioners in nursing* (pp. 238-261). Oxford, UK: Wiley-Blackwell.

Davis, K. (1999). Your attitude just might be my greatest barrier. *The Reporter, 4*(2), 1-3, 13. Retrieved from http://www.iidc.indiana.edu/index.php?pageId=466

Durand, V. M., & Merges, E. (2001). Functional communication training: A contemporary behavior analytic intervention for problem behaviors. *Focus on Autism and Other Developmental Disabilities, 16*(2),110-119.

Fouse, B., & Wheeler, M. (1997). *A treasure chest of behavioral strategies for individuals with autism.* Arlington, TX: Future Horizons.

Horner, R. H., Carr, E. G., Strain, P. S., Todd, A. W., & Reed, H. K. (2002). Problem behavior interventions for young children with autism: A research synthesis. *Journal of Autism and Developmental Disorders, 32*(5), 423-446.

Koegel, L. K., & LaZebnik, C. (2004). *Overcoming autism: Finding the answers, strategies and hope that can transform a child's life.* New York, NY: Penguin Books.

National Center for Learning Disabilities. *What is executive function?* Retrieved from http://www.ncld. org/types-learning-disabilities/executive-function-disorders/what-is-executive-function

National Institute of Mental Health. (2011). *A parent's guide to autism spectrum disorder.* Retrieved from http://www.nimh.nih.gov/health/publications/a-parents-guide-to-autism-spectrum-disorder/index.shtml

Schultz, W. P., & Searleman, A. (2002). Rigidity of thought and behavior: 100 years of research. *Genetic, Social and General Psychology Monographs,128*(2), 165-207.

Ylvisaker, M., Hibbard, M., & Feeney, T. (2006). *Flexibility versus rigidity in thinking and behavior.* Brain Injury Association of New York State. Retrieved from http://www.projectlearnet.org/tutorials/flexibility_vs_rigidity.html

Chapter 2:
The Problem

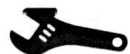

The first step of your behavior change program is to describe the specific problem, but this is not as easy as it seems. The description of the target behavior must be clear enough so that everyone will understand it and know exactly what to look for.

Let's examine the following statements:

- *She's disruptive.*
- *He lacks discipline.*
- *He's willful and controlling.*
- *He's oppositional.*
- *She never listens.*
- *He should know how to behave.*

Do you know exactly what the problem is by reading these statements? Not especially! Each of these statements can be interpreted in a multitude of ways. "She's disruptive" might mean that she takes toys from her siblings, or it could mean that she doesn't stay in her seat at dinnertime. We don't know what each statement means without more information. In fact, sometimes when adults describe a child or problems, we make erroneous assumptions and focus on our personal beliefs about the child, instead of describing specific problem behaviors.

The statements above may very well reflect how the child appears to the adult making them, but they do not give clear information about the child. They lack details to guide our actions. If we are going to develop successful interventions, it is crucial that problems be detailed in behavioral terms. This means that anyone who reads about the problem or listens to a description of it will understand the problem precisely. Describing the problem is not as obvious and simple as it seems. Here are some rules to guide you.

⚙ RULE: Be as specific as you can when describing the problem.

Let's talk about the statement *"He doesn't listen."* Usually, when parents make this statement, they mean, *"he doesn't do what I ask"* or *"he doesn't do what he's told."* They usually don't mean their child has a hearing problem. *"He doesn't listen"* isn't specific enough for anyone to decide how best to improve the child's "listening." It's hard to visualize what it means. We need to know more about the specifics. We need to know exactly what happens and when, as illustrated in the following.

Maybe your daughter runs away from you in the supermarket. Maybe your teenage daughter doesn't turn off the television when you ask her to come to dinner. Maybe your toddler hits your newborn whenever the baby cries. These circumstances are much clearer for us to "see." Most anyone can visualize a young boy running away from his mother in the grocery store, a teenage girl sitting in front of a television ignoring a parent, or a toddler hitting at a baby.

Let's review more examples of how to be specific in Illustration 2:1.

Illustration 2:1 Behavior Statements	
Vague Statement	**Specific Statements**
Won't share	Grabs stuffed animals away from sister.
	Takes all of the art supplies at the table.
	Pushes classmates out of the rocking chair.
Poor sport	Cries when he loses a card game.
	Screams when she can't have the red tokens.
	Quits before the ball game is over.
Is controlling	Tells siblings where to sit at the dinner table.
	Has to open and close the outside doors to the house.
	Pushes to be first in line.
Can't handle transitions	Protests when it's time to go to bed.
	Tantrums when it's time to turn off the computer.
	Lies on the floor when it's time to stop playing.
I can't take her anywhere	Won't stay with me in the store.
	Opens neighbor's cupboards when we visit.
	Won't keep her seatbelt on in the van.
He's always running off	Runs out of the classroom when he's upset.
	Doesn't come when I call his name.
	Hides from me in the park.
He won't keep his clothes on	Takes off her shoes and socks as soon as we are in the car.
	Takes his shirt off at preschool.
	Strips to his underwear as soon as we get home.
He's always breaking things	Drops glasses into the kitchen sink.
	Takes wheels off of little cars.
	Drops objects from the loft onto the floor below.
Tantrums	Cries and runs from the room.
	Screams, throws books, and calls people names.
	Hits his head against the wall.
Disruptive in class	Yells out math answers without raising his hand.
	Wanders about the room straightening things.
	Talks to his tablemates.
Poorly organized	Loses homework and planner.
	Isn't ready for the bus on time.
	Doesn't turn in work on time.
Noncompliant	Won't get dressed by herself.
	Won't turn off computer (television, music, electronic game).
	Refuses to do homework.

When you think about your child's behavior, be as specific as you can. Ultimately, this will make all of the problems more manageable. You may discover that problems share a common theme. For example, your child may argue about homework and avoid brushing his teeth. The common theme might be difficulties with fine-motor skills, such as writing and teeth brushing. Another common theme is a demand for predictability. For example your child might insist that you take the same route to school, fix him the same lunch every day, or that he wear the same pajamas to bed every night.

Sometimes parents discover that the child uses the same behavior in multiple situations. For example, the child has a tantrum at the store when he is told that he can't have a new toy, and he has a tantrum at home when it is time to eat dinner. He also has a tantrum at school when it is time for math. We talk more about the reasons for problems in the following chapters, but for now, let's practice making problems specific.

⚙️ To Do: Complete the problem statement practice: Illustration 2:2.

Look at the statements below. Put a ✓ in the box next to the statements that are specific enough for you to "see," and leave the boxes blank next to statements that are too vague.

   ☐ 1. My son takes all the fire trucks away from his classmates.

   ☐ 2. My daughter forgets to bring her books and planner to class.

   ☐ 3. My son is aggressive.

   ☐ 4. My daughter pulls her eyelashes and eyebrows out.

   ☐ 5. My son tells me to "shut up."

   ☐ 6. My son puts the Legos® away and shuts the closet door tight when cousins come to visit.

   ☐ 7. My son is oppositional.

   ☐ 8. My daughter won't put away the toys when she is done with them.

   ☐ 9. My son leaves homework at home.

   ☐ 10. My son never plays fair.

   ☐ 11. My son hits his face with his fist.

   ☐ 12. My daughter argues over everything.

   ☐ 13. My son gets upset when peers call him by his brother's name.

   ☐ 14. My daughter changes the television channel without asking first.

   ☐ 15. My son yells and throws the remote control to the TV.

   ☐ 16. My daughter doesn't write the assignments in her planner.

   ☐ 17. Everything has to be his way.

   ☐ 18. My son cheats so he can win the game.

   ☐ 19. My son won't compromise on which restaurant we eat at.

   ☐ 20. My daughter takes food from others' plates.

     Answers: Numbers 3, 7, 10, 12, and 17 are too vague and should be more specific.

Now that you have practiced identifying specific problem statements, the first tool for your Parenting Toolkit is the Daily Behavior Log.

✿ Tool: Daily Behavior Log

Illustration 2:3
Daily Behavior Log

Name: Josh   **Date:** April 4

Time	Activity	Behavior	Mood
7:00 a.m.			
7:15	Getting dressed	No problems	Happy
7:30			
7:45	Breakfast: cereal and milk		
8:00 a.m.			
8:15	Play with toys		
8:30			
8:45	Put toys away		Happy
9:00 a.m.	Computer		
9:15			
9:30	Turned computer off	Screaming for a few minutes	Angry
9:45	Car	OK	Calm
10:00 a.m.	Grocery store	Ran off in the parking lot	Laughing
10:15		OK in the cart	
10:30			
10:45		At checkout grabbing for candy, told no, crying	Upset
11:00 a.m.			
11:15	Car stopped in garage	Kicking back of my seat, fighting to get out of car	Angry
11:30			
11:45			
12:00 noon	Lunch: peanut butter and jelly sandwich, applesauce	Threw sandwich on the floor	Laughing
12:15			
12:30			
12:45	Nap		
1:00 p.m.			
1:15			
1:30			
1:45			Good mood

2:00 p.m.	At the park		Happy
2:15	Fed ducks		
2:30	Playing in the sand	Didn't want to leave; screaming, kicking	Angry
2:45		Dropping to the ground	
3:00 p.m.		Trying to get out of the stroller, crying	Upset
3:15	Home: snack	No problems	Calm
3:30	Cheese and crackers		
3:45			
4:00 p.m.	Speech therapy with Carol		
4:15			
4:30			
4:34			
5:00 p.m.	Car in the garage	Kicking back of my seat, fighting to get out of car	Angry
5:15			
5:30	Watching movie		
5:45	Turned off TV	Crying	Upset
6:00 p.m.	Dinner	Stuffed mouth with macaroni and cheese	Sad, upset
6:15		Had to remove bowl, cried	
6:30		Ate ice cream OK	Happy
6:45	Play	OK	
7:00 p.m.			
7:15	Clean up toys		
7:30	Bathtime		
7:45	Jammies/Potty/Teeth		
8:00 p.m.	Story		Happy
8:30	Bed		

Let's review the Daily Behavior Log example. It shows us that on April 4 this child screamed, kicked, and cried when the computer was turned off, when he could not have candy at the grocery check-out, when the car stopped in the garage (twice), when it was time to leave the park, when the television was turned off, and when his bowl was removed at dinner. We also know that he threw his sandwich on the floor at lunchtime and ran off in the grocery store parking lot.

Like a daily journal, The Daily Behavior Log is designed to record your child's daily activities, behaviors, and mood. It will help you accurately describe the problems so that you can effectively target a specific behavior for intervention. Using the Daily Behavior Log is fairly simple, whether you are experienced at record keeping or not. Simply begin to record your child's day in brief terms. Note when there are problems and when the day is going well. Focus on the specifics of the problems if you know them. Anyone with knowledge about your child's day should either tell you what happened or record it for you. Keeping the logs for a week or two is usually sufficient to get started.

Completing the Daily Behavior Logs for several days will tell us whether or not the same circumstances continue to produce the same or similar behaviors. Then we are ready to answer these very specific and important questions. If you are working with a professional, be sure to review your conclusions with her.

Using Illustration 2:2:

1. What are the behaviors you are concerned about? Be as specific as you can.

    Behavior A: *Running away in the parking lot*

    Behavior B: *Screaming, kicking, and crying*

2. When is the behavior most and least likely to occur?

    Behavior A – Most: *Any time we park in a large parking lot*

    Behavior A – Least: *If sleeping when we arrive*

    Behavior B – Most: *When told to turn off the computer or TV, told no, when has to leave park, car stopped in garage, bowl removed because playing with food*

    Behavior B – Least: *Getting ready in the morning, when playing; bedtime*

3. Where are the behaviors most and least likely to occur?

    Behavior A – Most: *At the grocery store, mall, or some other large parking lot*

    Behavior A – Least: *When at home or in a small parking lot*

4. With whom are the behaviors most and least likely to occur?

    Behavior A – Most: *With one adult*

    Behavior A – Least: *When there are two or more of us*

    Behavior B – Most: *Any adult*

    Behavior B – Least: *When alone*

The next step is to gather information to determine how extensive and severe a problem it really is. Review your Daily Behavior Log now and complete your Action Plan.

Action Plan for Chapter 2: The Problem
(Select From the Choices Below)

Rules to Remember:
☐ **Be as specific as you can when describing the problem.**

Tools to Use:
☐ **Daily Behavior Log**

To Do:
☐ **Problem statement practice: Illustration 2:2**
☐ **Describe the Problem:**
1. What is the behavior you are concerned about? Be as specific as you can.

2. When is the behavior most and least likely to occur?

    Most:

    Least:

3. Where is the behavior most and least likely to occur?

    Most:

    Least:

4. With whom is the behavior most and least likely to occur?

    Most:

    Least:

DAILY BEHAVIOR LOG

Name _____   **Date** _____

Time	Activity	Behavior	Mood
7:00 a.m.			
7:15			
7:30			
7:45			
8:00 a.m.			
8:15			
8:30			
8:45			
9:00 a.m.			
9:15			
9:30			
9:45			
10:00 a.m.			
10:15			
10:30			
10:45			
11:00 a.m.			
11:15			
11:30			
11:45			
12:00 noon			
12:15			
12:30			
12:45			
1:00 p.m.			
1:15			
1:30			
1:45			
2:00 p.m.			
2:15			
2:30			
2:45			
3:00 p.m.			
3:15			
3:30			
3:45			
4:00 p.m.			
4:15			
4:30			
4:34			
5:00 p.m.			
5:15			
5:30			
5:45			
6:00 p.m.			
6:15			
6:30			
6:45			
7:00 p.m.			
7:15			
7:30			
7:45			
8:00 p.m.			

References and Further Reading

Cohen, I. L., Yoo, H., Goodwin, M. S., & Moskowitz, L. (2011). Assessing challenging behaviors in autism spectrum disorders: Prevalence, rating scales, and autonomic indicators. In J. L. Matson & P. Sturney (Eds.), *International handbook of autism and pervasive developmental disorders* (pp. 247-270). New York, NY: Springer Science+Business Media.

Henry, S., & Myles, B. S. (2013). *The comprehensive autism planning system (CAPS) for individuals with autism spectrum disorders and related disabilities: Integrating evidence-based practices throughout the student's day* (2nd ed.). Shawnee Mission, KS: AAPC Publishing.

Horner, R. H., Sugai, G., Todd, A. W., & Lewis-Palmer, T. (2000). Elements of behavior support plans: A technical brief. *Exceptionality, 8*(3), 205-215.

O'Neill, R. E., Horner, R. H., Albin, R. W., Sprague, J. R., Storey, K., & Newton, J. S. (1997). *Functional assessment and program development for problem behavior*. Pacific Grove, CA: Brooks/Cole Publishing.

Chapter 3:

Is the Behavior Significant?

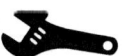

Think for a moment about your favorite activities; perhaps you watch television, surf the Internet, golf, gamble, play electronic games, or shop. Can these everyday activities ever become a problem?

Of course, they can. They are a problem if you engage in them exclusively, for long time periods, and with such intensity that they begin to interfere with your daily responsibilities and negatively affect those around you.

When we become so absorbed in our favorite interest that we miss work, forget about meals, don't get enough sleep, stop interacting with our families, avoid chores, and omit daily hygiene, there is a bigger problem. We assume our behavior is just fine, but those around us might disagree.

While the above activities are typically harmless, increasing the frequency, duration, and intensity can turn them into problems.

⚙ **Rule: Frequency, duration, intensity, setting, and persistence help determine the significance of a problem.**

In addition to the Rule of Five (see page 10), there are more aspects to consider when determining the significance of a problem. These include frequency, duration, intensity, the setting where a behavior is displayed, and chronicity. Let me explain.

Frequency – How Often Does Your Child's Behavior Occur?

Frequency refers to the number of times a behavior occurs in a time period, such as in an hour, a day, a week, or a month. Behaviors can occur once in a while or often. Think about a behavior like getting dressed. Most of us get dressed when we get up in the morning. Sometimes we change clothes after school or work. Usually, we change clothes again to get ready for bed. Changing our clothes 2-3 times a day in these circumstances is typically insignificant. But what if your child changes her clothes every time her shirt gets wet or dirty, or if she refuses to ever change her clothes, wearing the same shirt 24/7 for days on end? Now the frequency of the behavior (too much or too little) indicates a possible problem.

✅ To Do: Count and record.

To determine how often a behavior occurs, start to count every time you see it and keep track, either on a calendar or a chart. You can also use the Daily Log in Chapter 2 or the Weekly Behavior Log at the end of this chapter.

✳ Tool: Calendar

✳ Tool: Chart

✳ Tool: Daily or Weekly Behavior Log

You might be surprised to discover that behaviors you think happen "all the time" really only happen once or twice a day, or once or twice a week. Behaviors that occur once or twice a week are usually considered low in frequency, and some people might not consider them problems at all. Forgetting chores once or twice a week might not be significant, but missing the school bus twice a week could be significant. Problems that occur on three or more days a week are considered moderately significant whereas those that occur daily are severe and those that happen multiple times a day are extremely significant. Finally, behaviors that result in injury to self, others, or property are always significant, whether they occur once a month or once a day.

> *At all hours of the day or night 4-year-old Jack insists upon opening and closing the entrance doors to the house. When his father arrives home from work after midnight, Jack can hear the garage door open and runs downstairs to open the door into the house from the garage. He insists on letting the family pets in or out of the back door, opening the front door for visitors, and opening the door when he or any other family member or guest leaves. He is hyper-vigilant in his supervision of the doors and has a 20- to 30-minute meltdown if anyone else opens or closes a door. The frequency with which Jack opens and closes doors is extreme; it occurs multiple times a day. Jack has meltdowns for other reasons as well, typically because something does not go as he expects it to. The frequency of tantrums is 3-6 days per week, moderately significant.*

Duration – How Long Does Your Child's Behavior Last?

Duration refers to how long a behavior lasts. Some behaviors last a few minutes, while others can last for hours. Usually, the longer the behavior lasts, the more significant it is. Of course, there are exceptions, such as attention. Attention to task is one behavior where too short a duration, such as a few seconds, and too long a duration, such as hours, can both be significant.

✅ To Do: Measure duration by using a timer, clock, or a stopwatch.

✳ Tool: Timer

✳ Tool: Clock

✳ Tool: Stopwatch

Behaviors of less than 10 minutes' duration are usually mildly significant. Those that last 10-20 minutes are moderate, and those that last 20-30 minutes are considered very significant. Problem behaviors that persist for more than 30 minutes are extremely significant.

> *The duration of opening or closing a door is short; after all, it doesn't take long to do this. This behavior is mildly significant. Jack's tantrums last, on average, 20-30 minutes; therefore, his tantrums are considered very significant.*

Intensity – How Intense Is Your Child's Behavior?

Unlike frequency and duration, intensity is difficult to measure. Intensity is the power or force of a behavior. It can also be its strength.

✪ To Do: Think about the consequences.

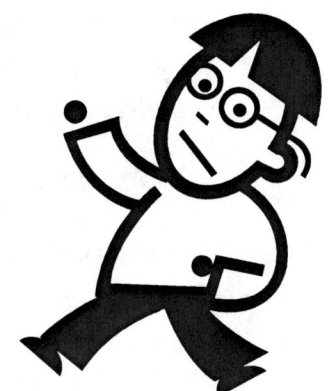

Determine intensity by thinking about the consequences of the behavior. The intensity of a tantrum can vary from mild crying to extreme rage and property destruction. Calling out answers in class in a normal voice volume can be mildly disruptive to the teacher and other students, but yelling them out can be very disruptive. Self-injurious behavior can range from slapping a leg with an open palm (mild potential for injury) to forcefully hitting one's head against a glass wall (great potential for injury).

> *Jack's passion for opening and closing doors is extreme, because under no circumstance can anyone else assume this task. The act itself is mild in intensity; he does not yank the doors open or slam them shut. When Jack is not allowed to open or close a door, he has a tantrum (the consequence). He screams, hits, and kicks family members, leaving bruises and marks on their bodies. This intensity of tantrum is extreme because it causes injury.*

Setting – Where Does Your Child's Behavior Occur? At Home? At School? In the Community?

The conventional environments for most children and teens are home, school, and community. Each setting presents opportunities for challenging behaviors to occur. Some children display problem behaviors in all settings, such as the child who pushes siblings at home, classmates at school, playmates at the park, and strangers at the mall. Other children display problems in one setting only, such as explosive behavior at school and not at home, or soiling at home but not at school. Some behaviors occur in multiple settings, but not all. For example, the child might have tantrums at home, at school, and in the community but never at her grandparents' home. Increased numbers of settings where behavior occurs also increases the significance.

In Jack's case, opening and closing doors does not occur any other place than home; therefore, this is mildly significant. However, Jack has tantrums at home, at preschool, in shopping centers, at restaurants, and at the park for a variety of other reasons. The multiple settings are considered extremely significant for tantrums.

Persistency – How Long Has Your Child's Behavior Been Happening?

Persistence is related to the Rule of Five, and refers to how long a behavior has been recurring. Is it well established? Has it persisted for weeks, months, or even years, or is it a relatively new problem? This information is important, because chronic, persistent problems are usually more difficult to change.

Jack has insisted upon opening and closing doors at home for six months. This problem is extremely disruptive to family life and, if it continues, will still be a problem in five months and five years. Tantrums have been occurring for two years. They are a chronic problem and will definitely be a problem in five years if they continue.

✿ Tool: Behavior Significance Scale

The Behavior Significance Scale (see page 29) is a tool to help determine the seriousness of the problem you are concerned about. It quantifies the variables of frequency, duration, intensity, setting, and persistence by having you score each from 1-4 (mildly to extremely significant). The final score will help you understand the total significance of the behavior – how severe the problem is and if intervention is needed now. The Behavior Significance Scale is a tool for your Parent Toolkit. Make multiple copies and score as many problems as you like (only one problem per scale). Later I will show you how to prioritize your list.

Using Jack's behavior as an example, Illustration 3:1 scores the behavior of opening and closing doors, and Illustration 3:2 scores tantrums. The scores are 4 + 1 + 3 + 1 + 3 = 12 for opening and closing doors. Notice that even though the duration and number of settings fall in the mildly significant range, the total score of 12 indicates a very significant problem. This number reflects the significant disruption this behavior causes the family and tells us that intervention is likely needed. Couple this with the score for tantrums (2 + 3 + 4 + 4 + 4 = 17), and we can understand that these are extremely significant problems.

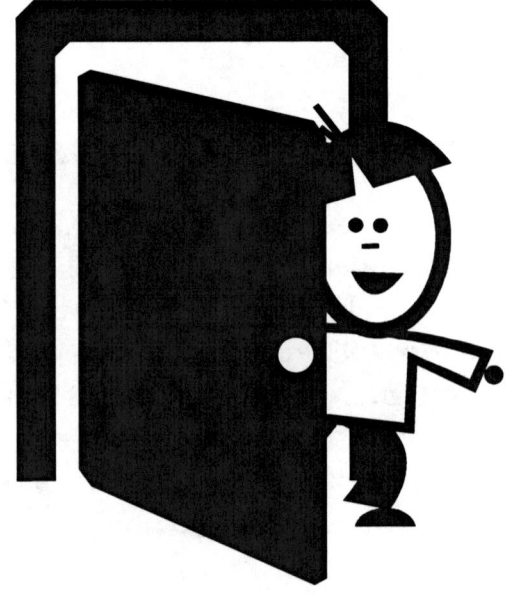

Illustration 3:1

Behavior Significance Scale – 1

Name: Jack_____   **Date:** April 12_____

Determine one behavior that you are concerned about and write it in the space below. Check one box in each row that best describes the behavior within the *past two weeks.* Write the number in the score column to the right. Add the numbers to obtain a total score.

Problem: Opening and Closing Doors_____

	1 **Mildly** **Significant**	**2** **Moderately** **Significant**	**3** **Very** **Significant**	**4** **Extremely** **Significant**	**Score**
Frequency *How often?*	0-2 days per week	3-6 days per week	Daily	Multiple times a day	4
Duration *How long?*	<10 minutes	10-20 minutes	20-30 minutes	> 30 minutes	1
Intensity *How intense?* *Consider the consequences.*	**Mild** Threatening, mildly disruptive	**Moderate** No injury, potentially dangerous/ illegal, disruptive	**Major** Minor injury, very disruptive	**Severe** People hurt, property destroyed, illegal	3
Setting(s) *How many?*	One	Two	Three	Multiple	1
Persistence *How persistent?*	< 1 month	1-5 months	6-12 months	> 1 year	3
				Total Score	12

1-5: Mildly significant
6-10: Moderately significant
11-15: Very significant
16-20: Extremely significant

Illustration 3:2

Behavior Significance Scale – 2

Name: Jack   **Date:** April 12

Determine one behavior that you are concerned about and write it in the space below. Check one box in each row that best describes the behavior within the *past two weeks*. Write the number in the score column to the right. Add the numbers to obtain a total score.

Problem: Tantrums

	1 **Mildly Significant**	2 **Moderately Significant**	3 **Very Significant**	4 **Extremely Significant**	**Score**
Frequency *How often?*	0-2 days per week	3-6 days per week	Daily	Multiple times a day	2
Duration *How long?*	<10 minutes	10-20 minutes	20-30 minutes	> 30 minutes	3
Intensity *How intense?* *Consider the consequences.*	**Mild** Threatening, mildly disruptive	**Moderate** No injury, potentially dangerous/ illegal, disruptive	**Major** Minor injury, very disruptive	**Severe** People hurt, property destroyed, illegal	4
Setting(s) *How many?*	One	Two	Three	Multiple	4
Persistence *How persistent?*	< 1 month	1-5 months	6-12 months	> 1 year	4
				Total Score	17

1-5: Mildly significant
6-10: Moderately significant
11-15: Very significant
16-20: Extremely significant

Illustration 3:3
Weekly Behavior Log

Sam							August 7- 13
Time	**Sunday**	**Monday**	**Tuesday**	**Wednesday**	**Thursday**	**Friday**	**Saturday**
7:00		Awake					Awake
7:15		Meds					Meds
7:30	Awake				Awake		
7:45	Meds			Awake	Meds		
8:00			Awake	Meds			
8:15			Meds				
8:30							
8:45						Woke him up	
9:00				Grocery store		Meds	
9:15				Chose cereal			
9:30				No wait		Dentist: OK	
9:45							
10:00	Church			Pet store		Social group	Grandma's
10:15	Stayed, drew,			Named fish		Did OK	happy
10:30	watched		Speech	Left OK	OT	Worked on	Swimming
10:45	clock		Worked hard	Used timer	silly	compromising	
11:00	**TANTRUM**			Gas station			
11:15	Wanted to go			(waited OK			
11:30	to McDonald's			with timer)			
11:45							
12:00		Camp	Camp	Camp	Camp		Lunch at
12:15							mall: OK
12:30						Pizza parlor	
12:45							
1:00	Bike Ride					Jake's party	Shoe Store
1:15	with dad					OK until	**TANTRUM**
1:30						opened gifts	No new shoes
1:45						Wanted to	left
2:00						keep the	
2:15						Lego® set	Wanted ice
2:30						**TANTRUM**	cream: "no"
2:45						Left early	**TANTRUM**
3:00	Did	Good camp	Good camp	OK camp	Hit camper at		Grandma's
3:15	good	Report (sub)	Report	Report	lunch		pool
3:30		computer	computer	computer	No computer		
3:45	computer				**TANTRUM**		
4:00		Sam visits					
4:15		Shares Legos®					
4:30		No fights !	Sets table				
4:45							
5:00							
5:15							
5:30	Dinner	Says bye!	Dinner				
5:45					Dinner		
6:00	Ride to	Dinner		Dinner			Wants to stay
6:15	airport					Dinner	in water
6:30	watched		Park	(Raining)			**TANTRUM**
6:45	planes		with bikes	Monopoly Jr			Dinner
7:00	OK when left		Played catch	not 1st!	Monopoly Jr	Sally's turn	
7:15	(used timer)		Swings	Able to leave	Lost game	to choose	
7:30			**TANTRUM**	unfinished		Movie	Went home
7:45			Wants to stay			**TANTRUM**	Tired
8:00					**TANTRUM**		Bed
8:15					Wants longer		
8:30	Bed	Bed	Bed	Bed	bath	Bed	Asleep
8:45			Asleep		Up until 10		

✿ Tool: Weekly Behavior Log

Similar to the Daily Behavior Log, the Weekly Behavior Log collects information about your child's activities and behaviors but over the entire week. It is a simple way to collect information about a specific behavior and the settings where it occurs. Nine-year-old Sam's parents collect information about his tantrums.

Looking at Sam's Weekly Behavior Log in Illustration 3:3, we see that he had a total of nine tantrums. This averages to more than once a day (even though on Day 1 he had no tantrums). Sam's Behavior Severity Scale is shown in Illustration 3:4. Totaling all of the scores, the severity rating score is 12, indicating a very significant problem.

Illustration 3:4

Behavior Significance Scale – 3

Name: Sam   **Date:** September 13

Determine one behavior that you are concerned about and write it in the space below. Check one box in each row that best describes the behavior within the *past two weeks*. Write the number in the score column to the right. Add the numbers to obtain a total score.

Problem: Tantrums

	1 **Mildly Significant**	2 **Moderately Significant**	3 **Very Significant**	4 **Extremely Significant**	**Score**
Frequency *How often?*	0-2 days per week	3-6 days per week	Daily	Multiple times a day	3
Duration *How long?*	<10 minutes	10-20 minutes	20-30 minutes	> 30 minutes	1
Intensity *How intense?* *Consider the consequences.*	**Mild** Threatening, mildly disruptive	**Moderate** No injury, potentially dangerous/ illegal, disruptive	**Major** Minor injury, very disruptive	**Severe** People hurt, property destroyed, illegal	2
Setting(s) *How many?*	One	Two	Three	Multiple	4
Persistence *How persistent?*	< 1 month	1-5 months	6-12 months	> 1 year	2
				Total Score	12

1-5: Mildly significant
6-10: Moderately significant
11-15: Very significant
16-20: Extremely significant

✅ **To Do: Use the Behavior Significance Scale.**

1. Complete one Behavior Significance Scale for each behavior you are concerned about. Discuss the scores with other family members if you would like or if you need more information before making a decision.

2. Tally the total scores for each behavior.

3. Record all the behaviors you have identified on a list, starting with the behavior with the highest score at the top and the lowest at the bottom (most significant to least significant).

4. Think about the Rule of Five and mark the behaviors that will definitely be problems in five years if they continue. (Those are the ones you will need to focus on soon.)

Where to Start

Remember the Rule of Five: **Behaviors that are problems now will likely remain problems in the future if there is no intervention.** These problems are significant and, therefore, require intervention. Start by concentrating on the areas that need the most attention right now rather than trying to address everything all at once. Some families begin with the behavior(s) that are causing the most disruption to family life. For now, choose one behavior that you want to think about as you read the rest of this book. Your goal is to come up with a plan that you can easily use after you have finished the book. Then you can go back and use the tools in your Toolkit for a different behavior. Who knows? Sometimes when we solve one problem, others start to be resolved, too.

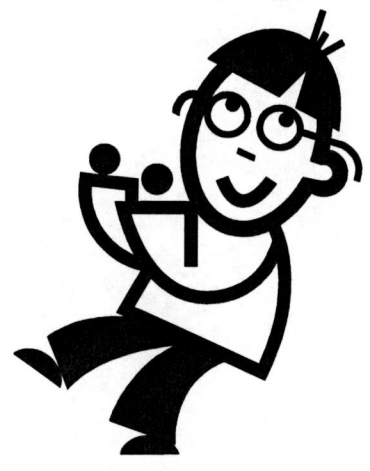

🗒️ Action Plan for Chapter 3: Is the Behavior Significant?
(Select From the Choices Below)

🔔 Rules to Remember:
☐ **Frequency, duration, intensity, setting, and persistence help determine significance.**

⚙️ Tools to Use:
☐ **Calendar**
☐ **Chart**
☐ **Daily Behavior Log**
☐ **Weekly Behavior Log**
☐ **Time, Clock, Stopwatch**
☐ **Behavior Significance Scale**

✅ To Do:
☐ **Complete the Behavior Significance Scale**
☐ **Total Score:** _____
☐ **The behavior is**
  ☐ **mildly significant**
  ☐ **moderately significant**
  ☐ **very significant**
  ☐ **extremely significant**

BEHAVIOR SIGNIFICANCE SCALE

Name: _____   **Date:** _____

Determine one behavior that you are concerned about and write it in the space below. Check one box in each row that best describes the behavior within the *past two weeks.* Write the number in the score column to the right. Add the numbers to obtain a total score.

Problem: _____

	1 **Mildly Significant**	2 **Moderately Significant**	3 **Very Significant**	4 **Extremely Significant**	**Score**
Frequency *How often?*	0-2 days per week	3-6 days per week	Daily	Multiple times a day	
Duration *How long?*	<10 minutes	10-20 minutes	20-30 minutes	> 30 minutes	
Intensity *How intense?* *Consider the consequences.*	**Mild** Threatening, mildly disruptive	**Moderate** No injury, potentially dangerous/ illegal, disruptive	**Major** Minor injury, very disruptive	**Severe** People hurt, property destroyed, illegal	
Setting(s) *How many?*	One	Two	Three	Multiple	
Persistence *How persistent?*	< 1 month	1-5 months	6-12 months	> 1 year	
				Total Score	

1-5: Mildly significant
6-10: Moderately significant
11-15: Very significant
16-20: Extremely significant

WEEKLY BEHAVIOR LOG							
Name:							Date:
Time	Sunday	Monday	Tuesday	Wednesday	Thursday	Friday	Saturday
7:00							
7:15							
7:30							
7:45							
8:00							
8:15							
8:30							
8:45							
9:00							
9:15							
9:30							
9:45							
10:00							
10:15							
10:30							
10:45							
11:00							
11:15							
11:30							
11:45							
12:00							
12:15							
12:30							
12:45							
1:00							
1:15							
1:30							
1:45							
2:00							
2:15							
2:30							
2:45							
3:00							
3:15							
3:30							
3:45							
4:00							
4:15							
4:30							
4:45							
5:00							
5:15							
5:30							
5:45							
6:00							
6:15							
6:30							
6:45							
7:00							
7:15							
7:30							
7:45							
8:00							
8:15							
8:30							
8:45							

References and Further Reading

Jang, J., Dixon, D. R., Tarbox, J., & Granpeesheh, D. (2011). Symptom severity and challenging behavior in children with ASD. *Research in Autism Spectrum Disorders, 5*(3), 1028-1032.

Oliver, C., McClintock, K., Hall, S., Smith, M., Dagnan, D., & Stenfert-Kroese, B. (2003). Assessing the severity of challenging behaviour: Psychometric properties of the challenging behaviour interview. *Journal of Applied Research in Intellectual Disabilities, 16*(1), 53-61.

Chapter 4:
Determining Why:
Reasons for the Behavior

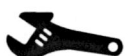

Tom's mother, Patty, is very frustrated because 15-year-old Tom does not take his shoes off when he comes into the house, despite numerous reminders, scolding, and reprimands. It is winter in the Midwest where they live, and this means snow and mud are tracked into the house daily. Tom won't wear boots to school (many teenage males don't), and he doesn't do a very good job of wiping his feet.

What is the problem? *Tom doesn't take his shoes off every day when he comes home from school. He is tracking mud and dirty snow into the house. This means more clean-up work for his mom.*

From Patty's point of view, Tom is "not listening." Remember our earlier discussion about listening in Chapter 2? She wonders why. Is he choosing not to take his shoes off because he is lazy, trying to upset her, or simply doesn't care about the extra work for her? Let's help Patty think about this problem in a new and different way.

⚙ Rule: Don't make assumptions: Gather facts.

When what we are doing is not working (in Patty's case, reminders, scolding, and reprimands), we need facts to help us figure out what is really going on. Without the facts, we can only guess. Sometimes that is OK, but most of the time guessing loses precious time and resources (like our sanity). It often takes children with autism a long time to learn a new skill or change behavior, so it is best to begin solving a problem with the most accurate information we can gather. Therefore, when a problem begins, become aware of the environment. Step back, listen, and watch; notice what is happening at the time.

⚙ Rule: Step back, listen, and watch.

Patty decides to watch Tom get ready for school. She discovers that it takes him many tries to tie his shoelaces and several minutes before he succeeds. She remembers that only recently he began to wear shoes with laces. (Lace-up athletic shoes are required for gym class, and the other high school teens don't wear shoes with Velcro®.) He tells her that once his shoes are tied for the day, he doesn't want to take them off again. It is much simpler to leave them on when he comes home, try to clean them as best he can, and endure her reprimands.

Patty now understands that Tom is not being willfully noncompliant, as she first assumed. Looking at the problem from a fresh perspective (Tom's point of view) and in a different way, she realizes that the real problem is that Tom has not mastered shoe tying. It takes him many attempts before he is successful. This is the real problem. Now all sorts of solutions become apparent.

What is the real problem? Tom has not mastered shoe tying.

Why didn't Tom just tell his mother that tying shoes was hard for him, especially after she started scolding him?

It is very typical for individuals with autism to assume that those around them have the same information as they do when, in fact, they don't. Tom takes for granted that his mother knows that tying shoe laces is hard for him, and he doesn't recognize that he needs to explain how hard and much trouble it is. He also doesn't recognize that he could ask her for help. He does not automatically understand Patty's point of view (tracking in dirt means more work for her) either. Even if she tells him, he may not comprehend that he must change his behavior (take his shoes off or explain why he cannot).

Misunderstandings such as this are typical in many problem situations. The solution is to observe, ask questions, and observe some more. We have to look at all facets of the problem and not just from our personal perspective!

Try not to take problems personally. Instead, look at the problem in a new and different way – **especially, the point of view of the person with autism.** Then you will have a greater chance of figuring out what the problem really is. With a verbal child, this is easier. When the child has limited language, your powers of observation become especially critical.

Often there are multiple reasons for a behavior, and primary, or root, causes are not easily identified. Identifying the many variables that make diverse and even cumulative contributions to the problem is like conducting a major investigation. So, think of yourself as a detective: observe, gather evidence, check, and record it. Your ultimate goal is to determine the potential reasons, or purpose, for your child's behavior and the variables that influence it. When you notice that a behavior is becoming a problem, start to observe and record information about what is happening at the time. As you do so, your description of the problem may change. You can start recording on the Daily and Weekly Behavior Log(s) at first, but you will need more specific information to determine the ultimate reason(s) for the problem.

✪ To Do: Collect and record detailed information.

Once you have chosen a specific behavior, record the circumstances every time the problem occurs. This gives you a wealth of information about the variables that possibly contribute to the problem.

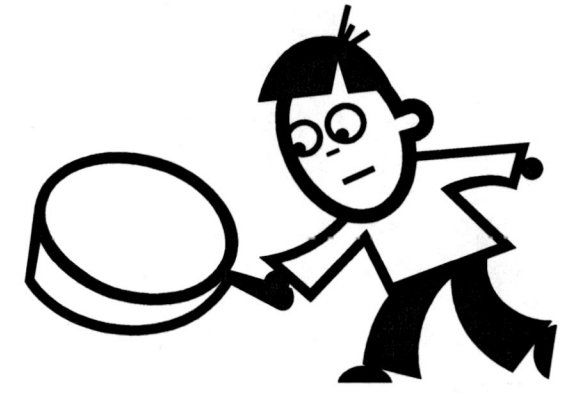

The more detailed you are in your information gathering and record keeping, the greater the likelihood you will be able to decode what is happening for your child at the time of the problem.

Tools to add to your Parenting Toolkit:

✿ **Tool: Problem Behavior Record**

✿ **Tool: Behavior Information Tool**

✿ **Tool: Sleep Chart**

Determine which tool is the best fit for your needs. In an ideal world, you will have a professional expert guiding you. These tools are most helpful when you have already identified a specific problem to solve. If you are still deciding what the problems are, continue to use the Daily or Weekly Behavior Logs in Chapters 2 and 3 to help you.

It is critical to find out why the behavior is occurring; therefore, make multiple copies of the tool of your choice and give them to anyone who interacts with your child who might encounter the problem you are recording. *Remember to look at the events from your child's point of view.*

✿ **Tool 1: Problem Behavior Record (Illustration 4:1)**

Start by filling in the behavior at the top, such as "Threw plate," "Bit sister," "Scratched mom," "Screaming," "Arguing over homework," etc. Fill in the date and time, and then check the boxes for the location, activity(s), triggers, presence of others, consequences, emotional states, environment, and health variables. The Problem Behavior Record can be completed quickly and easily. You simply check the appropriate boxes. It assists you in discovering patterns of behavior, a key to intervention.

> *Moriah, age 17, has no language and usually bites her arm when she is upset. Moriah is in the kitchen with her mother, Erica, setting the table for dinner. A quick survey of the environment indicates a noisy fan is on, tomato sauce is cooking on the stove, rolls are warming in the oven, and her brother is using the computer. It's cloudy outside, threatening to rain. Erica knows a thunderstorm is predicted for their area. She looks at Moriah's anxious face and sees her looking out the window. It is beginning to rain, and the sky is turning dark.*
>
> *Moriah starts to bite her arm. Biting her arm is one of Moriah's problem behaviors. Mother records the events on the Problem Behavior Record (Illustration 4:1). She is collecting data on the events that occur when Moriah bites her arm to determine any patterns. She has one clue today – a change in the weather. She will note weather changes in the future as she continues to record events.*

Illustration 4:1

Problem Behavior Record

Name: ___Moriah_____   Behavior: __Biting Arm_____

Date and Time: ___April 4, 5:30 p.m._____   Recorder: __Mom_____

Place: ☒ Child's Home   ☐ Other Home

☒ Kitchen   ☐ Child's Bedroom   ☐ Other Bedroom   ☐ Family/Living   ☐ Bathroom   ☐ Den/Office
☐ Basement   ☐ Garage   ☐ Yard   ☐ Hall/Foyer   ☐ _____

Other place:

☐ Vehicle   ☐ Small Store   ☐ Large Store   ☐ Restaurant   ☐ Fast Food   ☐ Park
☐ Office (appt.)   ☐ School Event   ☐ _____

Activity (at the time the behavior occurs):

☐ Dressing   ☒ Mealtime   ☐ Bedtime   ☐ Bath/Shower   ☐ Homework   ☐ Chore
☐ TV/DVD   ☐ Computer   ☐ Game system   ☐ Exercise   ☐ Project   ☐ Reading
☐ Writing   ☐ Music   ☐ Shopping   ☒ Watching   ☐ Playing   ☐ Talking
☐ Waiting   ☒ ___setting the table_____

Who is present when the problem occurs and what are they doing? Mom is making dinner, Sam is on the computer _____

Antecedent(s): What happened immediately before the problem?

☐ Given a Request/Demand   ☐ Request Denied   ☐ Difficult Task   ☐ Choice   ☐ Wait
☐ Mistake/Accident   ☐ Change in Activity   ☐ Interrupted   ☐ Conflict   ☐ Teased
☒ Unexpected Event/Surprise?   ☐ Disciplined/Reprimanded   ☒ ___starting to rain___

Child's emotional state immediately before the problem occurs:

☐ Calm/Relaxed   ☐ Happy   ☐ Frightened   ☐ Angry   ☐ Tired   ☐ Frustrated   ☒ Restless/Nervous
☐ Agitated/Irritable   ☐ Disappointed/Sad   ☐ Anxious/Worried   ☐ Overexcited/Overwhelmed

Adult's emotional state immediately before the problem occurs:

☐ Calm/Relaxed   ☐ Happy   ☐ Frightened   ☐ Angry   ☐ Tired   ☐ Frustrated   ☐ Restless/Nervous
☐ Agitated/Irritable   ☐ Disappointed/Sad   ☒ Anxious/Worried   ☐ Overexcited/Overwhelmed

Environment:

☒ Noisy   ☐ Quiet   ☐ Crowded   ☒ Hot   ☐ Cold   ☐ Windy   ☐ Cloudy   ☐ Sunny   ☒ Stormy   ☐ _____

Health variables:

☐ Thirst   ☒ Hunger   ☐ Pain   ☐ Injury   ☐ Illness   ☐ Medication change   ☐ Sleep change   ☐ _____

Why is it important to record my own emotional state?

Behavior is reciprocal. It goes back and forth, kind of like a game of tennis. The first person serves the ball (acts), and the other person hits it back (reacts). As adults, our emotions and how we react can inadvertently contribute to the problem. Some children mirror our emotions and reactions, while others become distressed when our facial expressions, tone of voice, etc., unexpectedly change. Your emotional state is an essential variable in the environment that also affects behavior.

Tool 2: Behavior Information Tool (Illustration 4:2)

The Behavior Information Tool uses a more open format than the Problem Behavior Record. This tool gives information about events that surround a behavior's occurrence. These events include the precursors (antecedents or A's), the behavior (B's), and the after effects (consequences, or C's). You record the antecedents and consequences of each episode of the behavior. Antecedents are the events that occur immediately prior to the behavior and ultimately give clues to the reason for the problem. Thus, antecedents are the precursors, what happens *before* the behavior does. Antecedents may be a setting, such as a restaurant; an action, such as being told no; an event, such as having to wait; volume, such as noise or shouting; or any other aspect of the situation that happens before the behavior. Be sure to write down specific antecedents, such as "We were at a party and Sarah dropped her bagel on her pants," or "Max was in the bathtub and I told him it was time to get out."

Antecedent ➡️ What happens first	Behavior ➡️ What happens next	Consequence What happens last
At a party, Sarah dropped her bagel on her pants	*Screaming*	*Went to the car until she was quiet*
In the bathtub, told Max time to get out	*Screaming*	*Ignored screaming and dried him off*

Consequences refer to what happens *after* the behavior. Consequences include your actions in response to the behavior, such as giving your child your attention, giving a warning, removing the child, ignoring, or giving the child what he wants. They also include ultimate outcomes – the final after effect – such as being rejected by peers, social isolation from family, or negative attention from classmates. The Behavior Information Tool allows you to write down your own impressions about the events.

> *Manuel, age 8, has multiple episodes of crying and screaming each day. His mother believes he cries "all the time." She starts to record the episodes on April 6 using the Behavior Information Tool (Illustration 4:2). Note that already there is a pattern of antecedents: he cries and screams in protest of her directions to come inside, eat spaghetti, do homework, and write sentences. All of these are clues to the reasons for the problem. After several more days, she should have a very good idea of the direction for her intervention.*

Illustration 4:2
Behavior Information Tool

Name: Manuel   **Date:** April 6

Behavior: Screaming, crying

Date/ Place	Time Began	Antecedent What happened immediately prior to the behavior?	Behavior	Consequence What happened immediately after the behavior?	Time Ended	Intensity (1-4)
4/6 Yard	5:30	Shooting baskets with Caleb; I tell him time to come inside for dinner	Screaming no, he wants to play more	Told him he could play 5 more minutes; Caleb goes home, M. sits outside alone	5:32	1
4/6 Table	5:45	Wanted a hamburger; I had made spaghetti; told him he had to eat some spaghetti	Screaming he wants a hamburger	Told him I would make the hamburger if he was quiet	5:55	2
4/6 Table	6:15	Wants to go back outside; I tell him he has to do his homework	Screaming no, he doesn't want to	I send him to his room; he cries and throws books; I say nothing	6:30	3
4/6 Table	7:00	Doing spelling homework; doesn't want to write words into sentences	Crying it's too hard	I write for him what he tells me; he stops crying	7:15	1

✿ Tool 3: Sleep Chart (Illustration 4:3)

Many children with autism have problems with sleep, such as settling into bed, sleep onset, co-sleeping (sleeping with a parent or another family member), restless sleep, frequent awakenings, or early morning awakening. The Sleep Chart is reserved for gathering information about such problems. Collecting specific information about your child's sleep habits will help you determine patterns of sleep, any environmental variables that might contribute to the sleep disturbance, and if she is a candidate for additional sleep study to help determine causes of the problems.

Illustration 4:3
Sleep Chart

Dates: _____ to _____   **Name:** _____

	7 8 9 10 11 12 1 2 3 4 5 6 7 PM AM	Naps	Comments
Sunday	/.........S_____UT_____A S_____A	1-3pm	Didn't want to go to bed

/ = In bed   S = Sleeping   A = Awake   UP = Urinated in pants   UT = Urinated in toilet

Naps = Time of any naps during the day   Comments: (environmental sounds, behavior)

✿ Tool Review

So far we have discussed several tools for your Parenting Toolkit. Here is a summary of what each is used for.

1. **Daily Behavior Log:** Use to identify multiple problems and decide upon a problem to start with. Record your child's behavior all day long, good and bad. This tool helps to determine when, where, and with whom problems are most and least likely to occur.

2. **Weekly Behavior Log:** Use when you have a good idea of the problem and are ready to collect data to determine how severe it is. It also gives you information about when the problem does NOT occur, which is useful for determining the reason for the problem.

3. **Behavior Significance Scale:** Use to determine how significant a problem really is; do you need to develop an intervention right now or is there another more significant problem?

4. **Problem Behavior Record:** Use to determine possible patterns for a single problem.

5. **Behavior Information Tool:** Use to record what happens before and after a specific behavior, the antecedents and consequences, so that you can reflect on possible reasons for it.

6. **Sleep Chart:** Use to gather information about your child's sleep habits.

At first, record keeping might seem time consuming and tedious. It is! But please do it anyway! Not only is this information critical to determining the correct intervention, it is necessary baseline information against which to measure any improvement, and the professionals who are guiding you will be able to help you determine the best course of action. Try to record immediately when the facts are fresh in your mind or as soon afterwards as you can. Reconstructing the information long after the behavior has passed increases the possibility for error.

✿ Rule: Behavior has a purpose.

Problem behaviors occur for a reason. Identifying those reasons often isn't easy and professional assistance is needed, but we must find them if we are to develop a successful intervention plan. Look closely at the information in your data records. Are there any obvious repeating themes or identifiable patterns? Does the same behavior occur in multiple circumstances? The pattern might relate to a time of day, event, person, or circumstance. When we start to notice themes, we are closer to discovering the antecedents that are highly probable causes or triggers of behavior problems. Then we can decide what action to take.

There are many reasons for human behavior. Some are obvious, like emotional reactions or a need for attention. Others are not so obvious but are very common, especially in children with autism. For example, a child may have multiple temper tantrums in a day; first in the morning because his favorite cereal is all gone (an unexpected event from his perspective); next when it is time for math class (to escape, protest because math is hard); he may have a third tantrum when he is last in line to the water fountain (his rule is that he is always first) and another one when his father is on the telephone (he wants help with homework). Here are four reasons for tantrums. Each reason requires a specific intervention plan. In this example, there is more than one reason for tantrums, and the same behavior (tantrum) is displayed in multiple circumstances.

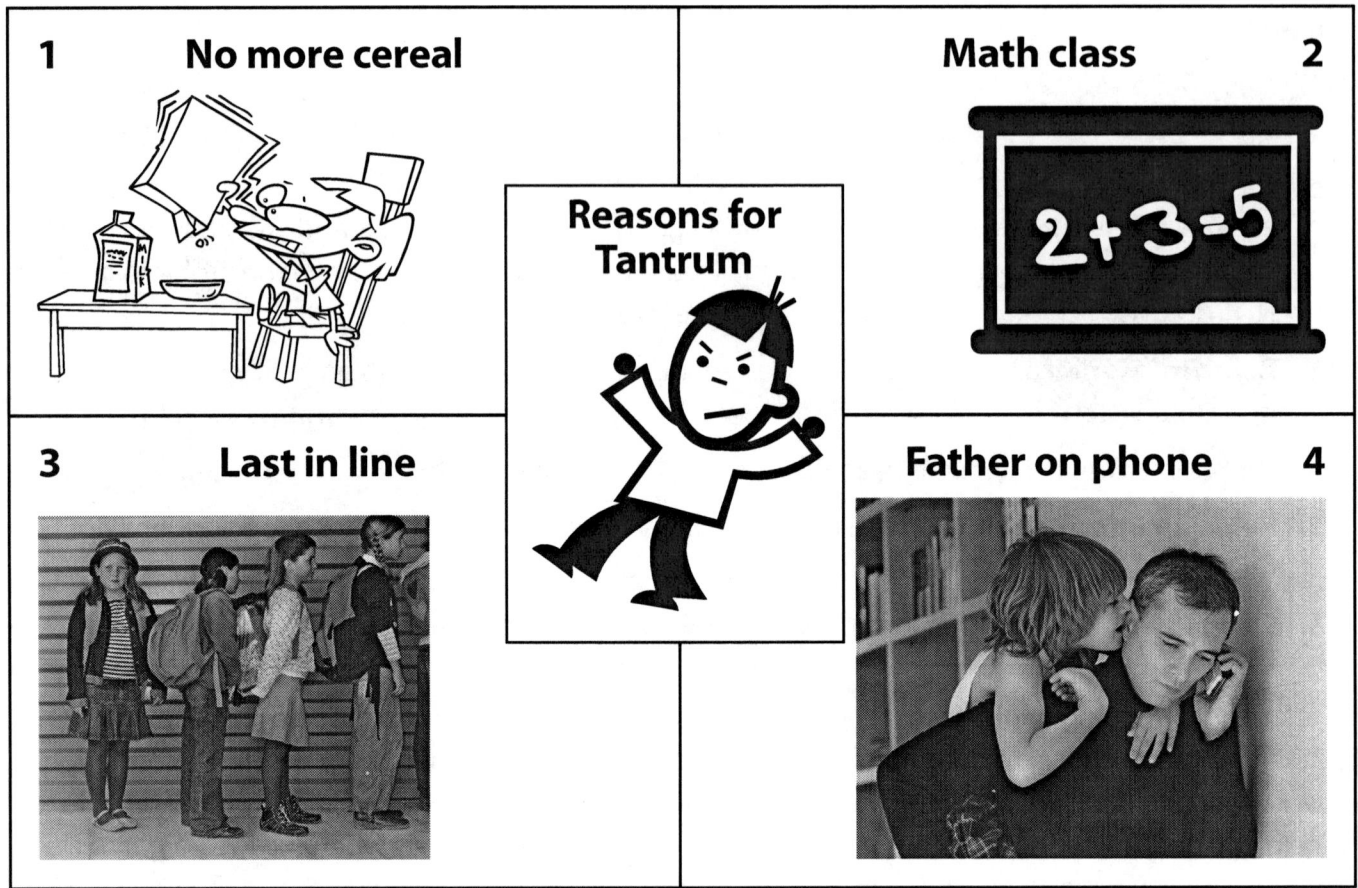

Multiple or different behaviors can serve the same purpose. For example, a child might wander away, ignore you, whine, scream, or hit as a way to protest the command to get ready for bed. Each night he might react with a different behavior to the same command, and on some nights use all of them. Each time the purpose is to tell you that he doesn't want to get ready for bed. Maybe because he doesn't want to stop playing, maybe because he is afraid of the dark, or maybe because he doesn't like to be alone. In each case, you need an intervention that addresses the transition to bedtime.

Sometimes the reason for a behavior is medical. Some children are unable to explain when they are in pain and may have a headache, ear infection, sore throat, dental abscess, urinary tract infection, or menstrual cramps. Any significant and unexpected change in a child's behavior should always be investigated for a possible medical cause.

Illustration 4:4 details possible reasons for behaviors. Take a look at it now and see what reasons might fit your child's behavior. Discuss your conclusions with the experts who are helping you, if any, then complete your Action Plan in this chapter.

Illustration 4:4 Possible Reasons for Behaviors	
Possible Reason for Behavior	**Such As:**
1. To escape, protest, avoid	☐ A demand or command or task ☐ A social situation ☐ Being refused or denied a request
2. To get or access something	☐ Attention. ☐ Help ☐ An object, treat, or activity
3. Need to change or transition	☐ Stopping a favorite activity in order to complete a non-preferred activity ☐ Stopping an activity that is unfinished ☐ Being interrupted ☐ Waiting ☐ Leaving ☐ Disruption in schedule or routine
4. Unexpected/unanticipated event/surprise	☐ Making a mistake on a task ☐ Being bumped or touched ☐ An unexpected sound such as a baby crying ☐ Receiving a lower grade ☐ Losing a game ☐ Substitute teacher ☐ Being told no or to stop
5. Knowledge or skill deficit: A difficult task, un-known rules, expectations	☐ Homework ☐ Daily chores/activities ☐ Social interaction skill ☐ Independent skill
6. Sensory overload: A challenging place (lights, noise, crowd, unclear expectations)	☐ Bus, school hallway, mall, restaurant, large store, cafeteria
7. Stressors/anxiety-provoking events	☐ Meeting new people, going to new places ☐ Family events ☐ Weather changes ☐ Specific fears (dark, monsters, needles)
8. Thoughts, rigid rules, obsessions, fixations	☐ "I always go first." "I always win." ☐ Fixation on a special topic or activity ☐ Miscommunication, misunderstanding, misinterpretation
9. Emotional reaction	☐ Fear, anger, anxiety, surprise, boredom, frustration
10. Medical: Relating to state of health	☐ Seizure ☐ Hearing/visual/motor impairment, ☐ Appetite, sleep, pain

Action Plan for Chapter 4: Determining Why: Reasons for the Behavior
(Select From the Choices Below)

Rules to Remember:
☐ **Don't make assumptions: Gather facts.**
☐ **Step back, listen, and watch.**
☐ **Behavior has a purpose.**

Tools to Use:
☐ **Problem Behavior Record**
☐ **Behavior Information Tool**
☐ **Sleep Chart**

To Do:
The possible reasons for my child's behavior are: _____

_____

_____

PROBLEM BEHAVIOR RECORD

Name: _____ Behavior: _____

Date and Time: _____ Recorder: _____

Place: ☐ Child's Home ☐ Other Home

☐ Kitchen ☐ Child's Bedroom ☐ Other Bedroom ☐ Family/Living ☐ Bathroom ☐ Den/Office
☐ Basement ☐ Garage ☐ Yard ☐ Hall/Foyer ☐ _____

Other place:

☐ Vehicle ☐ Small Store ☐ Large Store ☐ Restaurant ☐ Fast Food ☐ Park
☐ Office (appt.) ☐ School Event ☐ _____

Activity (at the time the behavior occurs):

☐ Dressing ☐ Mealtime ☐ Bedtime ☐ Bath/Shower ☐ Homework ☐ Chore
☐ TV/DVD ☐ Computer ☐ Game system ☐ Exercise ☐ Project ☐ Reading
☐ Writing ☐ Music ☐ Shopping ☐ Watching ☐ Playing ☐ Talking
☐ Waiting ☐ _____

Who is present when the problem occurs and what are they doing? _____

_____

Antecedent(s): What happened immediately before the problem?

☐ Given a Request/Demand ☐ Request Denied ☐ Difficult Task ☐ Choice ☐ Wait
☐ Mistake/Accident ☐ Change in Activity ☐ Interrupted ☐ Conflict ☐ Teased
☐ Unexpected Event/Surprise? ☐ Disciplined/Reprimanded ☐ _____

Child's emotional state immediately before the problem occurs:

☐ Calm/Relaxed ☐ Happy ☐ Frightened ☐ Angry ☐ Tired ☐ Frustrated ☐ Restless/Nervous
☐ Agitated/Irritable ☐ Disappointed/Sad ☐ Anxious/Worried ☐ Overexcited/Overwhelmed

Adult's emotional state immediately before the problem occurs:

☐ Calm/Relaxed ☐ Happy ☐ Frightened ☐ Angry ☐ Tired ☐ Frustrated ☐ Restless/Nervous
☐ Agitated/Irritable ☐ Disappointed/Sad ☐ Anxious/Worried ☐ Overexcited/Overwhelmed

Environment:

☐ Noisy ☐ Quiet ☐ Crowded ☐ Hot ☐ Cold ☐ Windy ☐ Cloudy ☐ Sunny ☐ Stormy ☐ _____

Health variables:

☐ Thirst ☐ Hunger ☐ Pain ☐ Injury ☐ Illness ☐ Medication change ☐ Sleep change ☐ _____

BEHAVIOR INFORMATION TOOL

Name: _____ **Date:** _____

Behavior: _____

Date/ Place	Time Began	Antecedent What happened immediately prior to the behavior?	Behavior	Consequence What happened immediately after the behavior?	Time Ended	Intensity (1-4)

SLEEP CHART

Dates: _____ **to** _____   **Name:** _____

	7 8 9 10 11 12 1 2 3 4 5 6 7 PM AM	Naps	Comments
Sunday			
Monday			
Tuesday			
Wednesday			
Thursday			
Friday			
Saturday			
Example	/.........S_____UT_____A S_____A	1-3 pm	Didn't want to go to bed

/ = In bed   S = Sleeping   A = Awake   UP = Urinated in pants

UT = Urinated in toilet

Naps = time of any naps during the day

Comments: (environmental sounds, behavior)

References and Further Reading

Aspy, R., & Grossman, B. G. (2007). *The Ziggurat model: A framework for designing comprehensive interventions for individuals with high-functioning autism and Asperger syndrome.* Shawnee Mission, KS: AAPC Publishing.

Cohen, I. L., Yoo, H., Goodwin, M. S., & Moskowitz, L. (2011). Assessing challenging behaviors in autism spectrum disorders: Prevalence, rating scales, and autonomic indicators. In J. L. Matson & P. Sturney (Eds.), *International handbook of autism and pervasive developmental disorders* (pp. 247-270). New York, NY: Springer Science+Business Media.

Davis, K. (1999). Your attitude just might be my greatest barrier. *The Reporter, 4*(2), 1-3, 13. Retrieved from http://www.iidc.indiana.edu/index.php?pageId=466

Fouse, B., & Wheeler, M. (1997). *A treasure chest of behavioral strategies for individuals with autism.* Arlington, TX: Future Horizons.

Meyers, S. M., Johnson, C. P., & the Council on Children with Disabilities. (2007). Management of children with autism spectrum disorder. *Pediatrics, 120,* 1160-1182. Retrieved from http://www.pediatrics. org/cgi/content/full/120/5/1162

Moskowitz, L. J., Carr, E. G., & Durand, V. M. (2011). Behavioral intervention for problem behavior in children with Fragile X Syndrome. *American Journal on Intellectual and Developmental Disabilities, 116*(6), 457-478.

Chapter 5

The Power of Antecedents

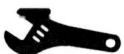

Changing the antecedents – the events that happen BEFORE the behavior – is an extremely powerful tool in your Parenting Toolkit. Sadly, it is often the last intervention adults think about when really it should be one of the first.

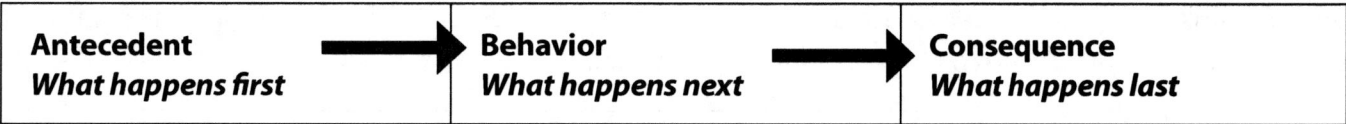

Antecedent *What happens first*	Behavior *What happens next*	Consequence *What happens last*

Antecedents are those events that happen right before the behavior occurs, such as a verbal command, a noise, or time of day, and give us important clues about the motivation for a behavior. When we have identified these events and, therefore, have a better understanding of the reasons for the behavior, we can intervene most effectively. Changing what happens BEFORE the behavior occurs may resolve a problem without any need for punishment or negative consequences. In fact, modifying the antecedents often prevents the behavior from happening in the first place!

Rule: Changing the antecedents – what happens before the behavior – often prevents the problem in the first place.

Before a behavior occurs is when we have our strongest influence. This is our best opportunity to stop problems from happening in the first place.

> *Melissa, age 6, has limited communication abilities, is very active, and has trouble sitting still. She is frequently reprimanded by the lunchroom monitors for getting out of her seat after she has finished eating while waiting for her class to be excused. Melissa loves to draw, so after getting permission from the teacher, her mother packs paper and crayons in Melissa's lunchbox, thus giving her something to do while waiting for her friends to finish eating. The activity is a huge success because, in addition to keeping her out of trouble, it encourages social interaction; she can share her paper and crayons with her friends and show them what she is drawing, and they can make comments about her drawings.*

When we only intervene **after** a problem occurs, such as with a reprimand, we will not succeed in permanently changing the behavior. Reprimands help adults feel better, but they do little to help the child with autism. We will discuss how to use consequences in later chapters. For now, we will concentrate on prevention. Let's learn more about the antecedents and how to use the Antecedent Checklist.

✿ Tool: Antecedent Checklist

The Antecedent Checklist lists multiple antecedents that may or may not have a direct effect upon your child's behavior. Remember each child with autism is unique. The list includes Environmental, Sensory, Communication, and Physical Variables, Required Skills, and Required Knowledge along with their definitions. The list is not comprehensive. Other antecedent variables may play a role in the problem and you may need professional help to confirm them. This list includes the key antecedents that are potentially within your control; those you might be able to validate and change.

In the example above, Melissa is out of her seat in the lunchroom after she has finished eating. The Antecedent Checklist in Illustration 5:1 shows us the variables that contribute to her behavior. Note that not all variables contribute. Those marked with a check mark are explained in boldface type. The others are left blank. This checklist demonstrates that multiple variables as well as lack of required skills and knowledge are contributing to Melissa's problem behavior.

	Illustration 5:1 **Antecedent Checklist – Melissa**	
Name: Melissa		**Date: 10/12**
Behavior: Out of seat		
	Environmental Variables	
✓	Setting	Place where the behavior occurs: **Lunchroom**
✓	Time of Day	When the behavior occurs: **Finished eating**
✓	Activity/Task	Activity at the time of the behavior: **Waiting for class to be excused**
	Materials	Any item used when the behavior occurs
✓	People	Persons who are involved in the behavior: **Melissa, lunch monitors, students**
	Sensory Variables	
✓	Auditory	Hearing (i.e., sensitivity to types of sounds or volume): **Lunch room noise**
	Temperature	The degree of heat, cold, a change in weather conditions
	Tactile	Relating to the skin and touch (e.g., texture of clothing, food, human touch)
	Olfactory	Sense relating to smells and interpreting odors
	Visual	Relating to sight
	Gustatory	Sense of taste/oral sensations from the tongue and taste buds (i.e., sweet, sour, salty, bitter)
	Vestibular	Sense of movement and maintaining balance
	Proprioception	Sense of body limb position in space (e.g., being able to drive a car without watching your feet or looking at the steering wheel)
	Communication Variables	
✓	Oral	Information a person can hear, use of verbal language: **Uses limited language**
	Visual	Information a person can see (e.g., a chart, list, photograph, object)
	Sign	Information a person can see through sign language
	Gestures	Information a person can see through body movements (e.g., a wave, shrug, nod)
	Augmentative	Alternative communication (an assistive device)

Physical/Biological Variables		
	Hunger	Change in diet, missed meals or snacks, change in eating habits, routine
	Thirst	Change in fluid intake
	Sleep	Change in sleep pattern, habits, or routine
	Illness	Presence of acute medical condition (e.g., infection, allergy symptoms, cold, flu
	Bowel Function	Presence of constipation, loose stools, change in bowel function
	Bladder Function	Change in urinary habits or routine
	Medication Effect	Change in medication, dose, administration time, missed dose
✓	Related Medical	Presence of chronic medical condition (e.g., seizure, hearing impairment; **ADHD**)
Required Skills		
	Fine Motor	Coordination required to control the smaller muscles of the body, such as for writing, fastening or playing an instrument
	Gross Motor	Activities that require large muscle groups (e.g., walking, running, sitting)
✓	Cognitive	Thought processes, reasoning, **problem solving, judgment**
✓	Social	Skills for interacting with and relating to others: **waiting, social conversation**
✓	Independent	Capacity to act without guidance from others: **mastery of waiting**
Required Knowledge		
✓	Expectations	The prescribed guide for one's actions, standard of conduct: **to remain seated**
✓	Rules and Routines	The principles and standards that guide actions: **lunchroom rules**
✓	Plans and Procedures	What is going to happen and how it is to be done: **waiting plan**
✓	Context	The circumstances where the skill or behavior is needed: **when finished eating**
Other		

By providing a specific activity in her lunchbox that is appropriate for waiting, we have addressed Melissa's need for required skills and knowledge; she now understands what to do after she has finished eating. Just telling her to sit and be quiet is not enough. Because of her attention deficit-hyperactivity disorder (ADHD) in addition to her autism and her limited use of language, Melissa has to be taught to do this. In addition, the activity becomes a means of fostering appropriate social interaction with her classmates. The need for reprimands is eliminated and, best of all, the problem is prevented from occurring.

Illustration 5:2 details the antecedents that contributed to Tom's situation (Chapter 4, refusal to remove his shoes). These include Environmental Variables, Required Knowledge, and Required Skills. Just as in Melissa's case, when armed with this information, the intervention has a different focus – teaching the skills necessary instead of punishing the behavior.

	Illustration 5:2	
	Antecedent Checklist Related to Tom's Situation	
Name: Tom		**Date: 4/10**
Behavior: Refusal to remove shoes at the door		
	Environmental Variables	
✓	Setting	Place where the behavior occurs: **home at the door**
✓	Time of Day	When the behavior occurs: **after school**
✓	Activity/Task	Activity at the time of the behavior: **untie shoes**
✓	Materials	Any item used when the behavior occurs: **shoes and laces**
✓	People	Persons who are involved in the behavior: **usually mother and Tom**
	Sensory Variables	
	Auditory	Hearing (i.e., sound sensitivity to types of sounds or volume)
	Temperature	The degree of heat, cold, a change in weather conditions
	Tactile	Relating to the skin and touch (e.g., texture of clothing, food, human touch)
	Olfactory	Sense relating to smells and interpreting odors
	Visual	Relating to sight
	Gustatory	Sense of taste/oral sensations from the tongue and taste buds (sweet, sour, salty, bitter)
	Vestibular	Sense of movement and maintaining balance
	Proprioception	Sense of body limb position in space (e.g., being able to drive a car without watching your feet or looking at the steering wheel)
	Communication Variables	
	Oral	Information a person can hear, use of verbal language
	Visual	Information a person can see (e.g., a chart, list, photograph, object)
	Sign	Information a person can see through sign language
	Gestures	Information a person can see through body movements (e.g., a wave, shrug, nod)
	Augmentative	Alternative communication (an assistive device)
	Physical/Biological Variables.	
	Hunger	Change in diet, missed meals or snacks, change in eating habits, routine
	Thirst	Change in fluid intake
	Sleep	Change in sleep pattern, habits, or routine
	Illness	Presence of acute medical condition (e.g., infection, allergy symptoms, cold, flu)
	Bowel Function	Presence of constipation, loose stools, change in bowel function
	Bladder Function	Change in urinary habits or routine
	Medication Effect	Change in medication, dose, administration time, missed dose
	Related Medical	Presence of chronic medical condition (e.g., seizure, hearing impairment)
	Required Skills	
✓	Fine Motor	Coordination required to control the smaller muscles of the body, such as for writing, fastening, or playing an instrument: **tie laces**
	Gross Motor	Activities that require large muscle groups (e.g., walking, running, sitting)

✓	Cognitive	Thought processes, **reasoning, problem solving, judgment**
✓	Social	Skills for interacting with and relating to others: **ask for help**
✓	Independent	Capacity to act without guidance from others: **mastery of shoe tying**
	Required Knowledge	
✓	Expectations	The prescribed guide for one's actions, standard of conduct: **untie and remove shoes at the door to keep floors clean and reduce work**
✓	Rules and Routines	The principles and standards that guide actions: **house rule is to remove shoes at the door**
✓	Plans and Procedures	What is going to happen and how it is to be done: **procedure for removing shoes, cleaning floors**
✓	Context	The circumstances where the skill or behavior is needed: **enter home**
	Other	

🔧 Rule: Teach skills instead of punishing behavior.

As we talked about in Chapter 1, negative behaviors don't self-correct and are not "outgrown." To change them requires a plan that often involves a different way of thinking coupled with creative parenting skills. After you have identified the specific problem and its antecedents, think about the appropriate behavior that you want from your child, instead of thinking about the negative behavior you don't want from your child. This is crucial to successful behavior change and solving problems.

🔧 Rule: Decide exactly what you want the child to do, not just what you don't want the child to do.

Let's go back to Tom. What are the positive behaviors we want to teach him?

1. Master shoe tying.

2. Wipe his shoes on a rug or mat.

3. Recognize when a task is difficult and ask for help.

4. Explain why he cannot do what he is asked to do.

5. Recognize that his actions have an effect upon other people and do something about it.

In reality, there are other problems in the course of Tom's day that relate to numbers 3, 4, and 5 above. Tom refuses to take out the garbage because he can't tie the bags securely closed, and he does not ask for help or explain why. This pattern of antecedents indicates that Tom's fine-motor skill challenges interfere with his ability to comply with parental expectations. However, his social and independent skill deficits (difficulty explaining why, asking for help, and recognizing the effect of his behavior upon others) also contribute to the problem.

Now that our thinking has shifted to asking why Tom isn't listening, the focus for intervention becomes teaching the skills and knowledge that he requires, instead of punishing him for "not listening." With support and guidance, he can make sustained progress and eventually achieve success in all of these problem areas, not just in tying his shoes.

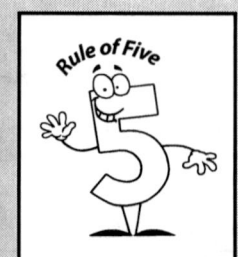

Rule of Five: Will this really matter? So what if he doesn't learn to tie his shoes?

I suppose Tom could wear slip-on shoes or shoes with Velcro® closures for the rest of his life, but he wants to be more like the other teens and chose to wear athletic shoes. So our job is to help him succeed. But more important, Tom needs help learning the effect his behavior has on other people, how to ask for help, and how to explain his actions. This is crucial if he is to succeed at work or in social interactions and relationships with others.

So, what can we do about the immediate problem of removing his shoes? Tom won't master these skills overnight. Here are some options.

1. First of all, stop punishing. Punishments can only be used after a child has mastered a skill, not before. (We talk more about punishment in Chapter 15.)

2. Buy new shoes for him that are easier to take off and put on. Slip-on or shoes with Velcro fasteners can be worn if he needs to go out again after school. This is his decision though, not the parents'.

3. Develop a reward system for removing shoes in the house (more about rewards in Chapters 8 and 9).

4. Set up 10-minute "tying practice" sessions and reward him for completing each session. He can practice with shoes, ropes, garbage bags, packages, etc. Once he can tie without mistakes, he might work against a timer to speed up his actions.

5. Add mopping the floor to his weekly chores. This will help him to appreciate the amount of work involved, learn a skill needed for independent living, and practice motor skills. Don't expect perfection, and give him an allowance for work done.

6. Finally, enlist the support of the teacher or occupational therapist. Perhaps opportunities to practice tying may also be found at school.

   Tom and his mother agree that the appropriate action for the immediate problem is for Tom to take his shoes off when he comes home from school. If he plans to go out later, he will wear athletic shoes without laces (the current fashion). Meanwhile, they will work on the skills of tying, asking for help, and answering why-questions.

✅ To Do: Review Antecedent Checklist.

Review the Antecedent Checklist at the end of the chapter and mark the antecedents that you surmise might have an effect upon the problem(s) that you are concerned about (one problem at a time). You may not be certain about some of the antecedents for a specific problem; put a question mark next to those that you are unsure about. If you are working with a professional, ask for guidance when selecting possible antecedents because this task is complex and can be confusing and overwhelming. Review your list of antecedents and think about those that you can change in an effort to positively impact your child's behavior.

Often, there are ways to reduce or prevent problems while you work towards more permanent solutions. For example, if your child doesn't like the sound of the vacuum cleaner, you can vacuum while she is at school. If she doesn't like the feel of woolen sweaters, buy her cotton ones. If she doesn't like bright light, use dimmer switches, change the window treatments, or have her wear sunglasses when outdoors. If she is sensitive to smells, use unscented cleaning or grooming products.

Most of these problems and their solutions create some temporary inconvenience for you and others in your family, but they don't interfere significantly with home life. But remember, most of them are short-term solutions. If we think about the Rule of Five, eventually you and your child will have to figure out more permanent ones; frequently under professional guidance and support.

Many other problems are not so easy to resolve, as illustrated below. Discovering their antecedents takes good detective work, time, and persistence.

Functional Analysis: Altering elements in the environment to see how behavior changes in a methodical manner is known as functional analysis. Typically planned and supervised by a highly qualified professional (such as a board-certified behavior analyst), a functional analysis is a systematic and purposeful approach to analyzing behaviors. By changing one variable at a time, you and the professional can determine the impact upon a child's behavior. This method is helpful when determining the reason for a complex problem, especially when a child has limited or no language. Although it is unwise for parents to conduct an experimental functional analysis without proper training and supervision, parents can observe their child, take data on behaviors as suggested here, and explore what is happening in specific circumstances.

For example, perhaps every night it is a struggle when your child is told to take a bath (or shower). Put yourself in your child's shoes and consider what is tough about taking a bath or shower. As illustrated below, many variables could be involved, so if your child can't tell you what the problem is, your job is to check out each possible one for the best explanation.

Problems Taking a Bath or Shower

Environment: Does the problem occur in any/all bathrooms or just one? Is there any time when bathing does not present problems? If so, what is different in those circumstances than in others? If your child does just fine at Grandma's, that is an important behavior clue to investigate. What is different at Grandma's house from your house?

Shower vs. bath: Is there a preference? If you don't know, try baths one week and showers the next. Some children prefer to sit in a tub full of water rather than having the water spray on them. For others it is the opposite – they prefer the constant temperature that a shower provides while baths can get cold.

Some of us prefer morning, others, evening bathing; is there a difference for your child? What about who is present in the bathroom with your child? Is there a difference in behavior with one or the other parent, or when someone else is present, like a sibling?

Sensory: Some children are bothered by the sound of the water hitting the side of the tub or the shower stall. Others don't like the constant spray that a shower provides, so a hand-held sprayer that they control helps, especially for washing hair.

The texture of the washcloth, sponge, or bath towel may contribute to resistance, or even the amount of pressure that the parent is using to wash or dry the child. Experiment with different textures and pressures.

Some children are afraid of soap and water getting in their eyes, nose, and mouth. A plastic visor on the forehead, goggles over the eyes, or using baby shampoo might help.

Temperature may change depending upon who is filling the bathtub or turning on the shower. Mark the faucet or the wall behind with a colored sticker so that everyone sets the same water temperature for several days. The smell of shampoo or soap might be the problem; you might try unscented products.

Finally, notice whether your child has trouble maintaining balance while standing in the shower.

Communication: How are you communicating to your child that it is time for a shower or bath? Are you interrupting a favorite activity? Are you giving sufficient time to transition? How do you communicate the steps in the bathing routine and the rules for expected behavior?

Physical/Biological Variables: Can you think of any physical or biological variables that might be persistently affecting the child's behavior?

Required Skills: This variable has to do with whether or not your child has the skills to complete an activity. How much help is needed? One question to ask is: Is this a "can't do" or a "won't do" problem?

"Can't do" problems are those for which the child needs to learn more knowledge and/or skills; a "won't do" involves any other of the antecedent variables.

Required Knowledge: Does your child know what is going to happen, the steps involved with the bathing routine? Does he know the rules, such as not to splash (keep water in the tub)? Does he understand the purpose of bathing or does he think it is time to play? When more than one person is involved, are your rules and expectations the same? The answers to all of these questions will help you sort out the cause(s) of your child's resistance.

There is a reason for the child's resistance to taking baths or showers. Once you have figured it out, you can modify the environment so your child is more comfortable. Is this really important? Yes! This is a problem that fits the Rule of Five. We want the child to master the independent skill of bathing. Children with autism have enough problems. We don't want to add more stigma because of poor grooming, a sure social turn-off.

By the way, once you figure out the reasons for your child's resistance and he is comfortable taking either a bath or a shower with your help, your next job is to teach him to wash himself. Look at Chapter 12 for strategies for teaching new skills.

This brings us to the next phase in our intervention planning. So far we have:

1. Identified the problem.

2. Determined the severity of the problem.

3. Identified possible antecedents and potential causes.

4. Begun to identify underlying variables that might contribute to the problem.

5. Started to modify antecedents.

Next, we will focus on communication and the tools for your Parenting Toolkit that are also essential to preventing problems in the first place.

Action Plan for Chapter 5: The Power of Antecedents
(Select From the Choices Below)

Rules to Remember:
- ☐ **Changing the antecedents – what happens before the behavior – often prevents the problem in the first place.**
- ☐ **Teach skills instead of punishing behavior.**
- ☐ **Decide exactly what you want the child to do, not just what you don't want the child to do.**

Tools to Use:
- ☐ **Antecedent Checklist**

To Do:
- ☐ **Review Antecedent Checklist**
- ☐ **Possible antecedents for the problem are:**
  - ☐ **Environment**　☐ **Sensory**　☐ **Communication**　☐ **Physical/Biological**
  - ☐ **Required Skills**　☐ **Required Knowledge**　☐ **Other**

ANTECEDENT CHECKLIST

Name:		Date:	
Behavior:			

		Environmental Variables	
	Setting	Place where the behavior occurs
	Time of Day	When the behavior occurs
	Activity/Task	Activity at the time of the behavior
	Materials	Any item used when the behavior occurs
	People	Persons who are involved in the behavior
		Sensory Variables
	Auditory	Hearing (i.e., sensitivity to types of sounds or volume)
	Temperature	The degree of heat, cold, a change in weather conditions
	Tactile	Relating to the skin & touch (e.g., texture of clothing, food, human touch)
	Olfactory	Sense relating to smells & interpreting odors
	Visual	Relating to sight
	Gustatory	Sense of taste/oral sensations from the tongue & taste buds (i.e., sweet, sour, salty, bitter)
	Vestibular	Sense of movement & maintaining balance
	Proprioception	Sense of body limb position in space (e.g., being able to drive a car without watching your feet or looking at the steering wheel)
		Communication Variables
	Oral	Information a person can hear, use of verbal language
	Visual	Information a person can see (e.g., a chart, list, photograph, object)
	Sign	Information a person can see through sign language
	Gestures	Information a person can see through body movements (e.g., a wave, shrug, nod)
	Augmentative	Alternative Communication; i.e. an assistive device
		Physical/Biological Variables
	Hunger	Change in diet, missed meals or snacks, change in eating habits, routine
	Thirst	Change in fluid intake
	Sleep	Change in sleep pattern, habits or routine
	Illness	Presence of acute medical condition (e.g., infection, allergy symptoms, cold, flu)
	Bowel Function	Presence of constipation, loose stools, change in bowel function
	Bladder Function	Change in urinary habits or routine
	Medication Effect	Change in medication, dose, administration time, missed dose
	Related Medical	Presence of chronic medical condition (e.g., seizure, hearing impairment, ADHD)
		Required Skills
	Fine Motor	Coordination required to control the smaller muscles of the body, such as for writing, fastening or playing an instrument
	Gross Motor	Activities that require large muscle groups (e.g., walking, running, sitting)
	Cognitive	Thought processes, reasoning, problem solving, judgment
	Social	Skills for interacting with and relating to others
	Independent	Capacity to act without guidance from others
		Required Knowledge
	Expectations	The prescribed guide for one's actions, standard of conduct
	Rules & Routines	The principles & standards that guide actions
	Plans & Procedures	What is going to happen & how it is to be done
	Context	The circumstances where the skill or behavior is needed
		Other

References and Further Reading

Aspy, R., & Grossman, B. G. (2007). *The Ziggurat model: A framework for designing comprehensive interventions for individuals with high-functioning autism and Asperger Syndrome.* Shawnee Mission, KS: AAPC Publishing.

Fouse, B., & Wheeler, M. (1997). *A treasure chest of behavioral strategies for individuals with autism.* Arlington, TX: Future Horizons.

Horner, R. H., Carr, E. G., Strain, P. S., Todd, A. W., & Reed, H. K. (2002). Problem behavior interventions for young children with autism: A research synthesis. *Journal of Autism and Developmental Disorders, 32*(5), 423-446.

Horner, R. H., Sugai, G., Todd, A. W., & Lewis-Palmer, T. (2000). Elements of behavior support plans: A technical brief. *Exceptionality, 8*(3), 205-215.

Meyers, S. M., Johnson, C. P., & the Council on Children with Disabilities. (2007). Management of children with autism spectrum disorder. *Pediatrics, 120,* 1160-1182. Retrieved from http://www.pediatrics.org/cgi/content/full/120/5/1162

Moskowitz, L. J., Carr, E. G. & Durand, V. M. (2011). Behavioral intervention for problem behavior in children with Fragile X Syndrome. *American Journal on Intellectual and Developmental Disabilities, 116*(6), 457-478.

Pratt, C., & Buckman, S. (1999). Supporting students with Asperger's syndrome who present behavioral challenges. *The Reporter, 4*(3), 6-10, 14. Retrieved from http://www.iidc.indiana.edu/index.php?pageId=467

Chapter 6:
Effective Communication

Now that you know the importance of antecedents – that is, of what happened before the behavior – for preventing problems, it's time to introduce a communication tool for your Parenting Toolkit. This tool is critical and should stay front and center in your Toolkit at all times. Miscommunication and misunderstanding are the root causes of multiple problems when parenting; therefore, changing to more effective communication is essential.

Deficits in communication and social behavior are core problem areas for children with autism. They don't have an innate ability to make and keep friends, to "fit in," or to work effectively with others. Their struggles in these areas are typically varied and life-long. All of their differences are unique. Some children have difficulties producing and using functional speech, while others recite movie dialogue, repeat comments or questions over and over, or lecture on special topics. Many have difficulties using gestures and facial communication effectively. All have difficulty understanding the ever-changing rules of social interaction and the perspectives of other people. Communication involves more than being able to speak. It also includes understanding.

Using Visual Communication

One very important characteristic of many children with autism is that they learn and retain information best when they **see it**, rather than hear it. This is called "visual learning," and the materials that are used to help this learning are called "visual supports."

What Is Visual Communication?

Visual communication, sometimes called visual support, refers to any information a person can see, such as a chart, a written list, a photograph, drawing, symbol, or picture. It can also be an object that means something, such as a ball representing time to play or a fork representing time to eat. Visual communication can also be a gesture, sign, or action; such as a hand motion that signals stop or come here.

Many of us program our destination into a GPS or Google the route in advance when planning a road trip. That's because we like to "see" where we are going and, turn by turn, know exactly how to get there. This also gives us a means to check and recheck the route if we need reassurance. The same is true for children with autism. They need such detail in order to know what to do, where to go, and how to get there. One way to communicate a new behavior expectation or rule is through visual communication. If you find yourself repeatedly and unsuccessfully telling your child the same thing, change your method of communication. The best choice may be visual communication.

> *17-year-old Meghan loves making movies on her laptop. She films scenes with her camera and then spends hours editing them into movies. This is her passion. However, her mother wants Meghan to help with daily chores, like folding and putting away the laundry. This is a task Meghan knows how to do well, but when she becomes absorbed in making her movies, she shuts out the world and doesn't want any interruptions. They argue, but Meghan ignores.*

> *Meghan has a driver's license, and her mother threatens to take away Meghan's driving privileges when she refuses to help. This "works" temporarily, but the next time Mother wants Meghan's help, they start arguing all over again. Both of them are frustrated and angry.*

> *During one of our sessions, I suggest to the mother that the next time she wants Meghan's help with the laundry, she write, "fold the laundry" on a sticky note and place it on the open laptop keyboard, right in front of Meghan, without saying a word.*

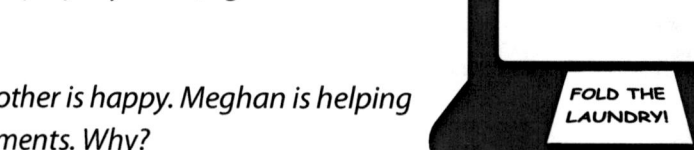

> *When I see them two weeks later, Mother is happy. Meghan is helping out, and there are many fewer arguments. Why?*

Most of us don't like to be interrupted when we are concentrating on something. The sticky note is not terribly intrusive, yet it clearly communicates what Meghan is expected to do. Writing out the expectation for Meghan is less intrusive than her mother's voice. It allows Meghan to pause her work at a place where she is comfortable. Also, the note is permanent, so Mother doesn't have to keep repeating herself. And most important, it helps both of them to stay calm.

⚙ Rule: Visual communication helps to communicate more effectively.

Effective for many, but not all children with autism, visual supports help to ensure that everyone has the same information. This includes knowledge of expectations and rules.

> *Michelle is a 12-year-old who loves to wear flip-flops, even in winter. When the weather turns cold, she and her mother argue every day about what shoes to wear. Michelle refuses to wear socks and sneaks flip-flops into her school bag. Her mother is concerned about frostbite from the often below-freezing temperatures.*

One cold day in November, Michelle enters my office wearing flip-flops. While she is getting her height and weight in an adjoining room, I ask her about her flip-flops, and she tells me she doesn't like to wear shoes. I suggest that perhaps we need a new rule. We return to my office, and I ask her mother to tell me the months of the year when it is OK for Michelle to wear flip-flops. She decides it is OK from April through October. When they leave, I ask them to write the rules on their calendar at home: April 1: "flip-flops." November 1: "put away flip-flops; wear boots or shoes." The next time I see Michelle, she shows me her feet and proudly says, "See my new boots."

Making an abstract rule such as "wear shoes when it's cold and in the winter" more explicit and adding it to the calendar helped Michelle to understand precisely what is expected.

Why Visual Communication Helps

There are many reasons why visual communication helps to moderate challenging behavior. They include the following.

✿ Rule: Visual tools help retain information.

Verbal communication is temporary and disappears once the words are spoken, but visual supports are stationary and can become permanent. They are a constant reminder of expectations, activities, schedules, rules, or routines. A visual tool such as a photo helps a child remember what you said and provides your child with a place to check if she forgets, doesn't understand, or wants reassurance. Visual tools help a child learn routines, such as the routine for checking in for an office appointment used by Jordan.

Jordan, age 15, uses a note card with the following text printed on it:

1. *Take out insurance card.*
2. *Take out blue hospital card.*
3. *Say: "Hello, I'm Jordan Jones. I'm here for my __ o'clock appointment with Judy Coucouvanis."*
4. *Give receptionist the insurance and hospital cards and wait for her to give them back to you.*
5. *Say, "Thank you."*

After Jordan has used the note card for a few visits, he decides he doesn't need it any longer because he knows what to do and can do it independently.

✿ Rule: Visual tools reduce the number of verbal directives needed.

How often do you find yourself repeating directions? Maybe you're not sure your child heard you, was paying attention in the first place, or was distracted by something along the way. As a result, perhaps you speak louder, with different words or more insistence.

An effective visual tool, such as a list, decreases the number of verbal directives and repetitions because both you and your child know exactly what is expected.

Mark, age 9, likes to bump down the stairs on his bottom, but his mother wants him to walk the "right way." She places multiple slips of paper in an envelope, some with " bump" written on them and most with "walk." Each time Mark is ready to go downstairs, he chooses a slip of paper and does what it says. Choosing becomes fun, is a distraction, and starts the day with everyone in a better mood. Mother gradually reduces the number of slips of paper with "bump" written on them. After a few weeks, Mark walks down the stairs the right way and doesn't need the envelope any more.

🔧 Rule: Visual tools highlight what is important.

Sometimes we give too much language too fast, and others can't keep up with us, especially if they have language disorders, hearing impairments, and are easily distracted. Visual communication, such as a schedule, focuses on what is most important without extra words or emotions. A schedule also provides your child with a place to check and recheck as often as he likes. Some children are experts at picking up details but miss the main point. But when key ideas, concepts, or expectations are presented visually, they are more apt to recall them.

🔧 Tool: Visual Schedule

A visual schedule helps children transition throughout the day by providing increased predictability and routine. Made from words, photographs, picture icons, magnets, or objects, it is a list that represents each activity or major transition. Visual schedules are especially helpful when your child has trouble with changes in routines. The schedule provides a predictable place to check what is going to happen that day so that he can better anticipate and mentally prepare for it, much like many of us check our personal planners. A schedule should not be static but reflect the actual events of the day. We want the child to learn that she can always determine what will happen next by checking the schedule. Many formats are available, including those you make yourself from photos or images when your child is young or cannot read or those you purchase, such as portable magnetic schedules or smartphone applications.

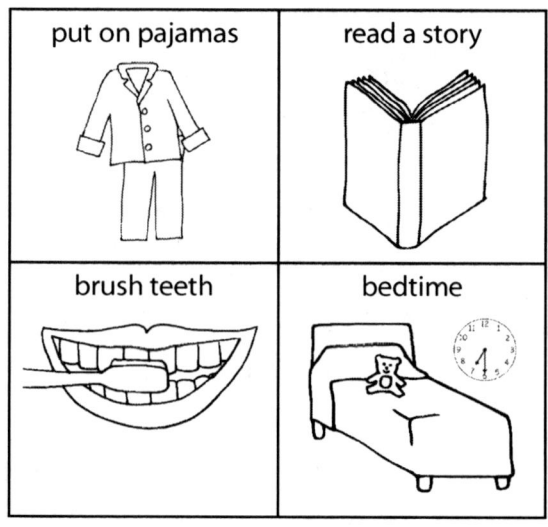

Schedules are typically used in school settings but are also helpful at home. A white or chalk board can give information about your schedule, such as "Gone shopping, be back around 8." Notes to your child can be used in these short-term circumstances also.

Many families place a large whiteboard in the kitchen (or use a desk-top-size calendar) and write in the schedule for the entire family – sports practices, therapies, sleepovers, appointments, non-school days, etc. It's a great tool for everyone, but especially for the child who fixates on the schedule. If your child can't read, use miniature picture icons.

AUGUST						
Sunday	Monday	Tuesday	Wednesday	Thursday	Friday	Saturday
10:00 Soccer ⚽ 1:00 Sam's birthday party 🧁	Alex dentist: 2:00	4:00 Soccer ⚽	6:00 School orientation 🏫		6:30 Dinner at café 👨‍🍳	1:30 Hair cut 💇 2:00 Shoe store 6:00 Grandma 👵

First and Then

Another way to show your child what is happening is to use a file folder with photographs of "First" and "Then." This type of schedule is very flexible and is especially useful when you take your child along on errands. Keep the folder and the photographs of the places that you visit regularly in your vehicle so they are ready when you need them.

Directions:

1. Use a file folder and write "First" on the front top left and "Then " on the front top right (see below).

2. Cut a slit in the front of the file folder in the lower-left side and label it "Finished."

3. Fasten an envelope to the left inside of the file folder over the cut.

4. Take photographs of your child engaged in daily routine activities.

5. Print the photos and fasten with Velcro® or a similar product to the inside of the file folder.

6. Attach the first activity to the front of the folder and sequence the next two or three activities on the right front side under "Then."

7. As each activity is finished, slide the photo into the 'Finished" slot and the envelope, then move the next activity into the "First" position.

8. Open the folder, select the next activity and place it at the end of the line of photos under "Then." For example, the next photo might be of the grocery store, or therapist, or anywhere the child is going in the car.

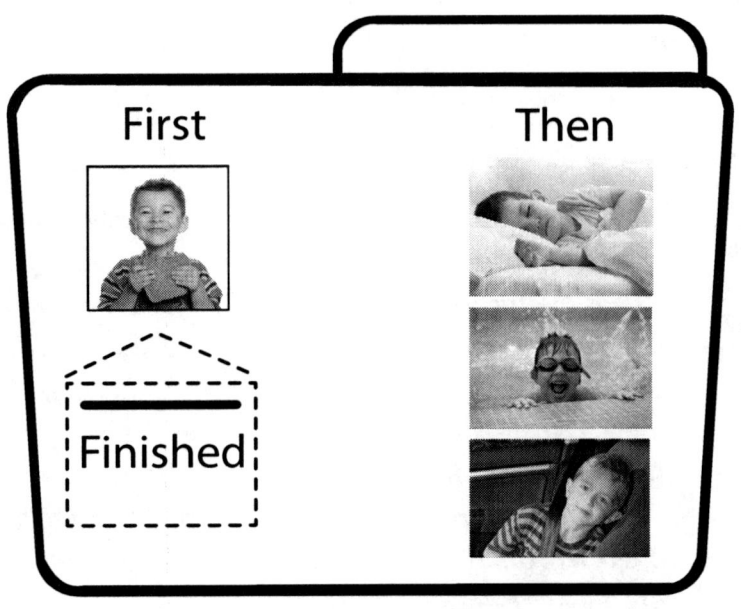

✪ Rule: Visual tools improve organization.

When we shop from a grocery list, our shopping becomes more structured and purposeful. Similarly, when a child completes daily chores from a list of expectations, the child can plan his time, secure in the knowledge that there won't be any surprises that might interrupt his favorite activities. Life becomes more predictable, and for some youth with autism, this is crucial to managing daily stressors. For example, a teenager might have a written checklist of daily after-school chores that must be completed by 6:30 p.m., such as:

☐ Set table

☐ Do homework

☐ Put away your laundry

☐ Empty dishwasher (put everything away in correct place)

☐ Get backpack ready for tomorrow

The teen can now plan his time, completing and checking off the tasks in the order he chooses. I will use more examples of visual tools in the remainder of this chapter and throughout the book. Remember that what works for one child may not work for another. Experiment with multiple formats, materials, and presentations to discover what works for your child. Be creative. There is no one right way!

Remember the saying "A picture speaks a thousand words." When your child sees what is expected, he may immediately understand and begin to do what you ask.

A simple task such as organizing a child's clothes can help him get ready in the morning.

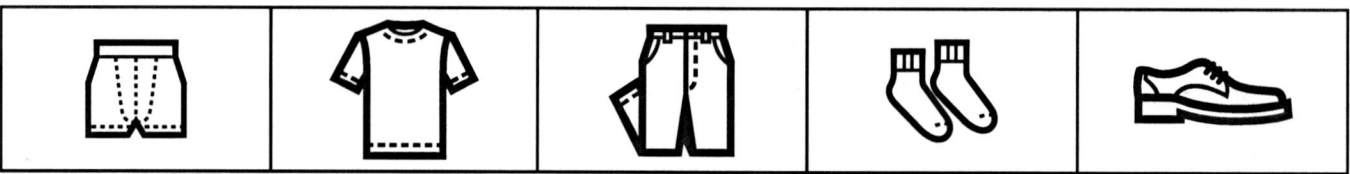

10-year-old Mary can't decide what to wear because she is never sure she has made the right choice, 8-year-old Sam is very active and has trouble focusing early in the morning, and 6-year-old Tricia wants to wear the same clothes every day. All three children benefit from having their clothes organized for the week ahead. Each has a special place labeled with the seven days of the week to keep each day's clothes, such as a hanging organizer, divided and marked shelf, or labeled baskets. A parent helps to choose one set of top, bottom, socks, and underwear for each day of the week and puts each set in its labeled place. When it is time to get ready in the morning, the child goes to the special place, retrieves that day's clothes, and puts them on. The visual labels and the special place help the child successfully and quickly get dressed every morning.

How do I know what type of visual support to use?

There are degrees of difficulty related to visual supports. The easiest to understand and use are real objects, followed by miniature objects of real objects, photographs of real objects, line drawings, symbols, and finally the written word. Here is the hierarchy of visual support to communicate ball.

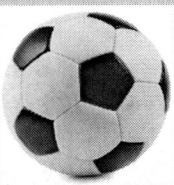
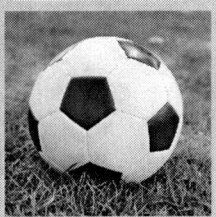
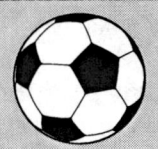

ball

Easiest ↑

1. Real object: Ball
   a. Requires very little interpretation
   b. Is useful for a very young child or somebody with significant developmental delay

2. Photograph of a ball
   a. Requires understanding that a three dimensional object can be represented by a two dimensional object

3. Drawing of a ball
   a. Requires understanding that the drawing represents any size or color ball

4. The written word "ball"
   a. Requires that a child is able to read.

Hardest ↓

How long do I keep using a visual tool? How do I know when my child doesn't need it any more?

That is kind of like asking an adult, "How long will you need your PDA, planner, or smartphone?" The answer is probably "a long time." Sometimes we decide a child "shouldn't" need the support any more, so we take it away. Do you know how lost many of us would be without our personal planners or PDAs? The same is true for children. Your child will let you know when he doesn't need the support any more. As long as he is using it, you should, too. As he ages, you may need to change the format (such as from a picture to a word) along with the expectation that he is to use it independently.

Parent Testimonial:

Our son, Alex, is a 17-year-old young man with autism. He has limited expressive language skills, but he can read simple words. Anxiety from not understanding what is required of him and/or not being able to express his needs and wants has led to behavioral issues.

Having access to a written schedule helps Alex to understand what is expected of him. It also helps him anticipate changes in his typical schedule. The written schedule helps him to understand where he will be during the week and gives him control over his days.

We start with a desk calendar that hangs in his room. At the beginning of the month, we pretty much fill every day with the known activities that will take place that month. These include school or home, therapies, appointments, and social activities like bowling or birthday parties. On Sunday evening, Alex likes to review his calendar with us and repeat what will be happening day by day during that week. He reviews whether he will be at school or home and who will be coming over during the week to help him, and what they will be doing. For example, "Monday, work, school, then home, 5:30 Sandy (his OT). Tuesday, school, then home, 5:00 Kelly (his tutor). Wednesday, school then home, Kari over (his sitter). Thursday, school, then home, 4:00 art class. Friday, school, then home, 5:30 bowling." By verbally reviewing his calendar and having it nearby for him to review he understands his week and can anticipate his activities.

This monthly desk calendar also helps Alex anticipate important changes in his schedule. He can look ahead and see when school starts or ends, when he will be on vacation, or when he may be taking a plane ride. He can anticipate doctor visits or activities that may cause him stress. Talking about it early and giving him the opportunity to understand what will be expected of him reduces his anxiety.

On a daily basis, we write on a 3x5 card his schedule of all the activities taking place that day. The card tells him where he needs to be, who he'll be with and, most important, that when the activity is over, he will be returning home. If I'm going to be out of the house, it tells him when I'll be returning home. One major benefit of the 3x5 card is that it is portable. Alex can carry it around with him during the day. (Many children with autism like to carry special things in their hands to reduce anxiety.) The card reduces Alex's anxiety during the day by giving him control and helping him understand his day.

If we are participating in an activity or visiting a place that may be confusing for Alex, we use a mini-schedule. This is written on another 3x5 card that details what we will be doing. As an example, when Alex used to visit the mall, he would walk in, get overwhelmed, and be ready to leave right way. He had no idea why we were there or what we were going to do. Now when visiting the mall, we write the stores we are going to visit on a 3x5 card and always end with having fries in the food court (a favorite activity). This lets him know where we will be going and offers him an incentive to be good while at the mall. If he misbehaves, our plan is to cross off fries and leave the mall; however, we have not had to do this. The schedule helps him understand all of our stops at the mall; he is fine being there now, so he always gets fries. We haven't had any behavior issues at the mall since implementing the mini-schedule.

By giving Alex a better understanding of his day/week/month, we have greatly reduced his anxiety. By having a better understanding of what will be required of him, he can anticipate his day and feel like he is in control of his schedule. This understanding has led to reduced anxiety and a significant reduction in behavioral issues.

Susan Weed

Using Verbal Communication

We spent time learning about visual communication first because it is usually very influential and a valuable problem solver. Now let's talk about using effective verbal communication. Remember that children with autism often have unique difficulties interpreting what you say. Many are very concrete and literal in their thinking. For example, idioms and metaphors, such as "I smell a rat," "Stop pulling my leg," "He took me to the cleaners," "Give him a big hand," or "Keep an eye out for her," are very confusing, and your child may not understand them.

Effective verbal communication techniques are often difficult for us to apply because they mean changing our behavior as parents in very specific ways. The focus is on our behavior, not the child's behavior. We get stuck in our behavior patterns, too. Let me explain.

Giving Directions, Commands, Demands

Parents typically give to their children two types of commands or directions. The first is a "start" command used when we want children to start to do something, like pick up toys, get dressed, or get ready for school. The next is a "stop" command, typically used when we want a child to stop an unacceptable behavior, such as hitting. Sometimes the two are combined, like when you want the child to stop playing and start to clean up or to stop watching a movie and start getting ready for bed. If your child has problems following your directions – whether you are giving start or stop commands – here are some rules to add to your Parenting Toolkit.

⚙ Rule: Be clear.

Be clear in your mind about what you want the child to do and why you want him to do it. Your request must be reasonable and one that he is capable of complying with. Use simple words. "We will go outside when you show me you are ready" is too vague. "Ready" must be defined. "We will go outside when you have your coat on" gives more information. "First coat, then outside" is even simpler.

⚙ Rule: Get the child's attention.

Be sure you have the child's full attention. Remember he has communication problems and may not fully understand every word you say. So to ensure success, go near him. Don't yell from a neighboring room. You may need to say his name and have him look towards you before you speak; that's OK. In fact, teaching him to respond to his name by looking towards the speaker shows he is listening to what is being said, a good social skill to develop.

⚙ Rule: Be positive.

Being positive can be difficult when your own feelings are getting in the way. Watch your voice tone and volume. State what needs to be done and avoid challenges. Try not to act upset or angry. Many children with autism learn from what they see, so modeling appropriate, calm behavior can help, whereas angry behavior does not. So if you can't be happy and upbeat, at least try to be calm and matter-of-fact in both your voice tone and volume. Turning your directive into a game, a contest, or some other fun activity is one way to be positive. For example, set a timer and see if your child can finish the task before the timer rings.

⚙ Rule: Make the last word count and eliminate contractions

Choose your words carefully. Use clear, concise, and simple words. The last word you say is often the most important, so make it count. "Don't do that" is not an effective command. It does not give enough information. "That" – the last word – gives no direction to your child whatsoever. In addition, contractions are difficult to understand so try not to use them either. When you use a contraction, often the last words are prompts to do exactly what you do not want the child to do. Think about the request "Don't throw the toy." The last words, "throw the toy" prompt the child to throw the toy. Instead, drop the contraction and tell the child exactly what you want him to do, "Give it to me. Put it on the table." Then the last word you say may prompt the correct action. If your child finds some food on the floor and picks it up with the intention of eating it, "Don't put that in your mouth" or "Don't eat it" will probably invite the very action you are trying to prevent. A more effective response is "Throw that in the garbage" or "Dirty, leave it on the floor."

⚙ Rule: Slow things down. Reduce your language.

Constant repetitions of directions teach children eventually not to listen to the words. Multi-step and complex instructions are usually overwhelming and confusing, and frequent repetition of directions only teaches the child that the adult does not mean the direction the first time.

When your child isn't listening to you, try to figure out why. Perhaps you are using too many words and speaking too quickly. Simplify your language and be specific. Tell your child exactly what you want him to do. For very young children, two to three words are often best, especially when teaching a new behavior or skill (i.e., *stand up, come here, coat on*). These words must replace the commands, demands, or threats being used before. See Illustration 6:1.

Illustration 6:1
Giving Directions

Instead of saying …	**Say …**
Come back.	*Sit down.*
Get ready to go.	*Put on your shoes.*
Stop eating with your fingers.	*Use your fork.*
Stop picking.	*Put your hand in your pockets.*
Aren't you listening to me? Don't touch.	*Sam, look. Hands down.*
Don't run.	*Please walk.*

🔩 Rule: Tell the child what you want him to do (instead of what you don't want him to do).

When you determine exactly what you want your child to do (rather than what you don't want her to do), everyone in the life of the child understands what is acceptable to say and what is expected of the child. Everyone should use the same word(s) to avoid confusing the child; therefore, consider what is easiest for your child to understand and for others to remember. For example, the new phrase, such as "hands down" or "quiet voice," becomes the command or directive. If you emphasize the inappropriate behavior, such as "don't hit, don't push" or "don't scream," no one knows exactly what the child is supposed to do instead, **including your child**.

🔩 Rule: Prompt BEFORE the unacceptable behavior happens.

When you anticipate a problem, prompt your child before the unacceptable behavior occurs. For example, if you think your child is going to hit his sister, say "Hands down," "fold hands," "hands to yourself," or "high five." Any of these proactive statements tells him exactly what to do and may prevent hitting.

> ***Why can't I say, "Don't hit!" or "No hitting!"?***
>
> These words don't give any new information and could inadvertently prompt bad behavior. Think about "please don't hit" or "no hitting." If these are the only words you use, the last word is "hit" or "hitting," a prompt to do just that.

🔩 Rule: Use "real" choices.

Avoid questions with a choice unless the child really has a choice and you are ready to accept "no" as an answer. When you say, "time for bath, OK?" or "can you put your coat on?," you are giving the child the choice to say "no." If it really is time for bath, simply say, "time for bath."

If your child protests when you give a verbal direction, offer a different choice with the same end result, such as, "Time for bath, are you going to take your duck or the penguin to swim with you?" "Time to put your coat on. Are you going to do it by yourself or with my help?" "Time to clean up. Are you going to start with the blocks or the trains?" Give the child some time to think about the choice. You may also need to repeat the last few words, "blocks or trains?" Giving choices in this manner can be an effective distraction and gives the child some control – he gets to make the ultimate choice, and yet your demand is met also.

🔩 Rule: Use specific, not general, time references.

Phrases such as "in a while," "later," or "in a few minutes" are too general and abstract for most young children with autism to understand. It is hard to know what "in a while" means. Give the child a specific time reference, such as "after school," "before bed," "on Sunday morning." "First … then" or "When … then" phrases can help, too. "*First* put on your pajamas and brush your teeth, *then* we will read a story." "*When* you eat your cereal, *then* you can go play." To speak even simpler, say something like, "*First* cereal, *then* play."

⚙ Rule: Add extra information.

Add extra information when the child does not start to do right away what you ask. This is the time to show your child what to do or to add visual tools, such as a schedule or a photograph. When you use a schedule say, "check your schedule" before giving the direction. The schedule tells the child what to do so you don't have to. In fact, if you use a schedule, try not to tell your child what is next. The goal is for the child to look at the schedule and then start to do the activity without you, thus creating independence. Instead of telling, point to the next activity if you think an extra prompt is needed. If your child still doesn't comply, then you can add verbal directions.

A typical mistake is to add extra information by offering an explanation, such as "put your coat on because it is cold outside." Rather than complying, some children argue with the explanation, "It's not cold outside." Ask the child to repeat the direction, tell or show the child exactly what to do, and praise compliance.

"Put the crayons in the box" is a specific direction. If the child does not comply, extra information would be to add a visual cue by modeling the direction, picking up one of the crayons while repeating, "putting the crayons in the box," and then showing the child what to do and putting the crayon in the box.

⚙ Rule: Don't give a directive if you don't have time to follow through.

One of the biggest mistakes parents make is not following through. (This is true for parents of typically developing children as well!). Inadvertently, some of us teach our children NOT to listen to us. When we repeat directives multiple times and then give up and either do the task ourselves or let it slide until later, our children learn that our words don't really mean anything. They learn to ignore what we say. Obviously, we're not intentionally teaching our children to ignore us. We get interrupted, the phone rings, we have to go to work – any number of life events get in the way of our follow through.

Try not to give the directive in the first place if you don't have time to follow through. This fundamental rule is essential to teaching compliance. If you don't have time to ensure the toys are put away before a therapy appointment, leave them until you return. If you have to get to work and your child hasn't taken out the garbage, leave it. Deal with it when you get home. When your goal is to teach your child to listen to what you say, then you have to be the one to follow through, no one else.

⚙ Rule: Praise and reward compliance.

We will talk more about praise and rewards in Chapter 8. The important message here is that when you are trying to teach your child to do what you ask, praise and rewards can help. Let your child know you appreciate her efforts and reward her successes.

⚙ Rule: Practice.

Learning to use these rules and tools takes practice, and individual family members are often in prime positions to coach each other's performance. Gentle reminders from your spouse when you say "OK?" at the end of a direction or "don't" will help you recognize and change your behavior. Genuine words of encouragement and sincere feedback help everyone to develop new communication skills. Calmly review problem situations after the fact and incorporate everyone's ideas and suggestions to ensure all the right steps are in place for the child. Set aside some time to practice using these verbal communication tools and ask your family to review your performance.

One tool for giving directions that I frequently share with parents is presented in Illustration 6:2.

Illustration 6:2
Tool: Giving Directions

1. Make sure you have time to follow through.

2. Think through what you are going to say and do.

3. Get the child's attention; state his name.

4. Give the direction, wait, and silently count slowly to 5 (may repeat once).

5. Repeat the direction using the same words and add extra information, such as a gesture, hand signal, or visual tool.

6. Praise immediately when the child starts to comply.

7. If he does not comply, make a decision:
    – Model what to do (e.g., start to pick up the toys).
    – Offer a real choice.
    – Physically guide the child to start. Always use the minimum amount of physical contact necessary for the request to be completed. Don't praise!
    – Praise when he starts the next step/task independently.

8. Never complete the request by yourself, but follow through later if needed.

When we can communicate exactly what we want the child to do, with visual supports and with words, we have mastered one of the most helpful rules of parenting a child with autism and – believe it or not! – the child is more likely to do what we ask.

Armed with our new communication tools, let's move on to the next step in changing behavior – how to make and use rules, one of the hallmark challenges facing parents of children with autism.

Action Plan for Chapter 6: Effective Communication
(Select From the Choices Below)

Rules to Remember:
- ☐ **Visual communication helps to communicate more effectively.**
- ☐ **Visual tools help retain information.**
- ☐ **Visual tools reduce the number of verbal directives needed.**
- ☐ **Visual tools highlight what is important.**
- ☐ **Visual tools improve organization.**
- ☐ **Rules for giving directions, commands, and demands:**
  - ☐ *Be clear.*
  - ☐ *Get the child's attention.*
  - ☐ *Be positive.*
  - ☐ *Make the last word count and eliminate contractions.*
  - ☐ *Slow things down. Reduce your language.*
  - ☐ *Tell the child what you want him to do (instead of what you don't want him to do).*
  - ☐ *Prompt BEFORE the unacceptable behavior happens.*
  - ☐ *Give "real" choices.*
  - ☐ *Use specific, not general, time references.*
  - ☐ *Add extra information.*
  - ☐ *Don't give a directive if you don't have time to follow through.*
  - ☐ *Praise and reward compliance.*
  - ☐ *Practice.*

Tools to Use:
- ☐ **Visual Schedule**
- ☐ **Visual Supports/Tool(s)**
  1. _____
  2. _____
  3. _____
- ☐ **Giving Directions Tool (Illustration 6:2)**

To Do:
- ☐ **The Communication Plan is:** _____
  _____
  _____

References and Further Reading

Bernard-Opitz, V., & Häußler A. (2011). *Visual support for children with autism spectrum disorders: Materials for visual learners*. Shawnee Mission, KS: AAPC Publishing.

Brereton, A., & Broadbent, K. (2007). *Helping young children to communicate using visual supports* (ACT-NOW Fact Sheet 26). Melbourne, Australia: Monash University, Centre for Developmental Psychiatry & Psychology. Retrieved from http://www.med.monash.edu.au/spppm/research/devpsych/actnow/download/factsheet26.pdf

Cardon, T. A. (2007). *Initiations and interactions: Early intervention techniques for parents of children with autism spectrum disorders*. Shawnee Mission, KS: AAPC Publishing.

Fouse, B., & Wheeler, M. (1997). *A treasure chest of behavioral strategies for individuals with autism*. Arlington, TX: Future Horizons.

Hodgdon, L. A. (1995). *Visual strategies for improving communication, Volume 1: Practical supports for school and home*. Troy, MI: QuirkRoberts Publishing.

Hodgdon, L. A. (1999). *Solving behavior problems in autism: Improving communication with visual strategies*. Troy, MI: QuirkRoberts Publishing.

Koegel, L. K., & LaZebnik, C. (2004). *Overcoming autism: Finding the answers, strategies and hope that can transform a child's life*. New York, NY: Penguin Books.

McClannahan, L. E., & Krantz, P. J. (1999). *Topics in autism: Activity schedules for children with autism; Teaching independent behavior*. Bethesda, MD: Woodbine House.

Quill, K. A. (Ed.). (1995). *Teaching children with autism: Strategies to enhance communication and socialization*. New York, NY: Delmar Publishers, Inc.

Chapter 7:

Teaching New Rules

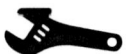

Rules govern what all of us say and do. There are rules for social interaction, rules for public behavior, mealtime rules, rules when we visit family or friends, rules for school, rules for worship, rules for driving, rules for playing games – rules for just about any situation you can imagine. Some behavior challenges involve misunderstanding the rules.

The Hidden Curriculum

Most youth with autism like to know the rules. In fact, when the rules are explicit and predictable, they usually follow them (and often tell others the rules, too). The trouble is that rules change, depending upon the situation and the circumstances. Most typical children grasp these changes without too much difficulty. For example, they quickly learn that rules for eating in a restaurant are different from rules for eating at home, which are different from the rules for eating at a friend's or relative's house, which are different from eating at a picnic or at a ball game. But all these different rules are bewildering and overwhelming for many youth with autism because they are not able to instinctively figure them out and cannot automatically relate the rules they know to new situations. Sometimes these unspoken rules are referred to as the "hidden curriculum." This term refers to the rules that we and others, often in error, assume your child knows. These rules are usually unwritten and include the dos and don'ts of everyday actions. Your job is to help your child learn the rules, remembering that you will have to teach in multiple situations.

Replacement Behavior and New Rules

The next step to changing a behavior, or solving a problem, is to figure out the rules that your child will need to learn to apply in the appropriate circumstances. However, in order to make the rules explicit for your child, you have to make them explicit for yourself first.

Alicia, age 12, has limited language. She and her mother, Yazminn, often visit their neighbor. Alicia likes to explore the various rooms in their neighbor's house, including closets and cupboards, while Yazminn chats with her friend. Yazminn is embarrassed and distressed by Alicia's behavior. Sometimes she scolds her and tells her to sit down, at other times she makes excuses for her, hoping that her neighbor will understand. However, she realizes that if the wandering continues, Alicia will not be welcome. In their culture, visitors sit quietly and talk to each other.

In this example, the problem is that Alicia is wandering, uninvited, throughout the neighbor's home. Identifying what she is supposed to do instead is the first step in helping her learn the rules for visiting. In this case, her mother wants her to sit quietly. This behavior, sit quietly, is called the "replacement behavior;" it "replaces" wandering, which is the problem behavior in this situation.

> *However, Yazminn has been telling Alicia to sit down all along and, therefore, concludes that this expectation is clear. So why doesn't Alicia comply? Yazminn completes the Antecedent Checklist (see Chapter 5) and decides that Alicia does not have the skills and knowledge to entertain herself while visiting friends. She is unable to carry on a reciprocal conversation and is probably bored during these visits. She doesn't know what to do with herself.*

🔧 Rule: Sometimes the expected behavior is not as obvious to the child as it is to you.

Even though your child "knows" not to do something, she may not know exactly what to do instead. So you have to define and teach the new rules and expectations.

> *Yazminn decides to bring one of Alicia's favorite books or photo albums with her so that Alicia has something to do while Yazminn is talking to her friends.* **The Rule is: Sit quietly and look at your book.**

🔧 Rule: Everyone involved must know the new rule(s).

This "new" rule replaces the "old" problem behavior of wandering. Voicing the rule is critical, because everyone who interacts with the child in similar circumstances must be absolutely clear about the new expectations. They must use the same language and consistently follow the plan. Think about a way to communicate the replacement behavior and the new rule to others.

> *Yazminn develops a rule card to help Alicia (and others) remember the rules for visiting. On the front is a picture of Alicia sitting appropriately. On the back, it says: 1. Don't walk around the house. Stay in your seat. 2. Fold your hands and sit quietly. 3. Look at your book.*

> *When Alicia follows the rules, she earns a special sticker when they return home. When they first start using the rule card, they make their visits short so that Alicia can experience success.*

It is typical for several people to be involved in any child's life. Each may have personal ideas about appropriate rules and behaviors, and each may be telling or doing something different. For youth with communication deficits, such as autism, this adds to the youth's confusion. So, it is essential to get everyone on the same page, including the child.

⚙️ To Do: Determine the replacement behavior: Practice Activity 7:1.

Look at the examples of problem behavior below. Pick one replacement behavior for each problem behavior. The replacement behavior that you select becomes the "new rule," which is communicated to the child using the phrase "the rule is …" In Practice Activity 7:1, the first replacement behavior is completed for you. The language used for the rules can be simple or more complex, depending upon the child's communication skills. For example, if there are too many words in the first example for your child, the new rule might be simply to "trade."

This task might seem strange, especially since you don't have more information about the context or the reasons for the behavior in the first place. But the purpose is to demonstrate that there is no magic to determining new rules for your child; in fact, some rules will be quite obvious to you. The key is to create very specific rules that make the expectations and circumstances more predictable for your child and help everyone else understand the rules, too.

This type of activity helps to prepare you and your child for the skill of problem solving. In future chapters, we discuss that often there is more than one correct solution, or rule, but your child doesn't understand that. You will have to teach him one rule at a time. Remember, rules are what you want your **child to do instead** of the problem behavior. Possible answers to Practice Activity 7:1 are available at the end of this chapter.

Practice Activity 7:1: Determine the Replacement Behavior	
Current Problem Behavior	**Replacement Behavior = New Rule for the Child: "The new rule is . . ."**
Grabs stuffed animals away from sister.	Trade stuffed animals with your sister when you want hers.
Pushes brother out of the rocking chair.	
Cries when he loses a card game.	
Cheats so that he can win the game.	
Tells siblings where to sit at the dinner table.	
Pushes to be first out the door.	
Cries and screams when it's time to get ready for bed.	
Cries and screams when he can't buy something in the store.	
Won't stay with me in the store.	
Won't keep her seatbelt fastened in the car.	
Runs out of the classroom when she's upset.	
Hits his head against the wall when he's frustrated.	
Takes off her shoes and socks as soon as we are in the car.	
Insists we always eat at Big Boy.	
Fully tears book pages that have a little tear.	
Isn't ready for the bus on time.	

Why don't the new rules include words like "no," "don't," or "not"?

When the replacement behavior is "don't hit your head on the wall," it doesn't tell the child (or anyone else) what to do instead. It is crucial that we define the "instead of" for any problem that involves harm to self, others, or property. So instead of "don't hit your head on the wall," we might decide, "take a break," "get your Vantage" (communication device), "squeeze your hands," or "sit in the red rocking chair."

For a child who hits a baby who is crying, the new rule cannot be "no hitting" or "don't hit." We need to decide exactly what we want the child to do instead. Choices might include "get mom or dad," "get a pacifier for the baby," "cover your ears," "turn on music," etc. Then all of us know what the child is supposed to do *instead of* hitting, and we can work together in multiple situations to teach him the new rule.

You can include rules with "no" or "do not" in special circumstances *after* you have defined the replacement behavior; then both can be used. See Isaac's Rules on page 87.

When we can articulate exactly what we want the child to do, we have mastered one of the most helpful rules of parenting a child with autism – and – the child is more likely to do what we ask.

Is there anything else to consider when choosing a replacement behavior or making a new rule?

The replacement behavior must be doable, meaning that your child must have the skills needed to perform it. It must also be possible to achieve and must be logical, practical, and realistic given the circumstances. Sometimes we determine a replacement behavior that we truly believe is achievable for the child; however, after we develop and use the intervention, we discover we are off base. For example, you might decide that your child should trade toys with others, but then discover that he doesn't know how to give a toy to someone else. This is perfectly normal. Simply revise the plan to include an alternative behavior that is achievable.

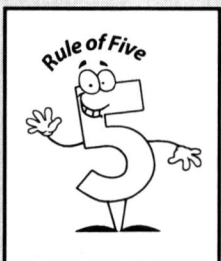

Finally, think about the future. Will the new behavior continue to be appropriate as your child ages? We spend the majority of our lives as adults, not children, so give youth the tools they need to be successful and as self-reliant as they can be in adulthood. Ask, "Will this new rule still be acceptable in five months, five years?" If the answer is yes, then you have identified an appropriate replacement behavior. If the answer is no (or maybe), choose something else.

Mary Beth, age 9, insists upon a different bedtime routine every night. The routines keep getting longer and longer so it's taking up to two hours for her to settle into bed. This seriously affects her ability to get up in the morning and ready for school, creating significant conflict between her and her parents. In addition, she is often overtired when she arrives at school, which affects her ability to concentrate. If this problem continues, it will definitely be a problem in five months and five years. The reason for the problem is likely obsessive thinking and anxiety about bedtime.

Mary Beth's parents agree that a reasonable expectation for a bedtime routine is 30 minutes. Given past experience with their daughter, they know that she is capable of settling down within 30 minutes. Settling for sleep within 30 minutes fits the Rule of Five because it is a reasonable expectation as Mary Beth gets older.

However, they also realize that their daughter will need help to accomplish this. Part of the problem is the ever-changing bedtime routines. Sometimes she wants her mother to put her to bed. Sometimes her father does it. Sometimes she wants three stories, sometimes four stories, sometimes a movie, etc. Some nights she takes a bath, on others she does not. Her parents realize more predictability and consistency is needed. All of them need to be on the same page.

They enlist Mary Beth's help and decide upon three different, yet reasonable, bedtime routines. The routines are written step by step on note cards and placed in an envelope. Each night, at bedtime, they say to Mary Beth, "The rule is: Choose a card, ready for bed in 30 minutes." Mary Beth chooses a card from the envelope and follows the routine presented.

When Mary Beth follows her rule, she receives a special treat in her lunchbox the next day. If she is successful all week, she earns a special activity on the weekend.

Determining a new rule is just one tool for your Parenting Toolkit. Let's look at more tools for how to explain and teach rules to your child.

Visual Communication

Visual supports are used to teach new rules. They **show** a child appropriate and inappropriate behavior – "use a tissue," "keep your hands in your pockets," "keep your clothes on," or "use a quiet voice" can all be expressed visually with a photograph, drawing, or written list. These new rules replace "don't pick your nose," "don't put your hands in your pants," "don't strip," and "don't yell." Notice the difference? The negative phrases don't tell your child what to do. The new rules tell your child exactly what to do!

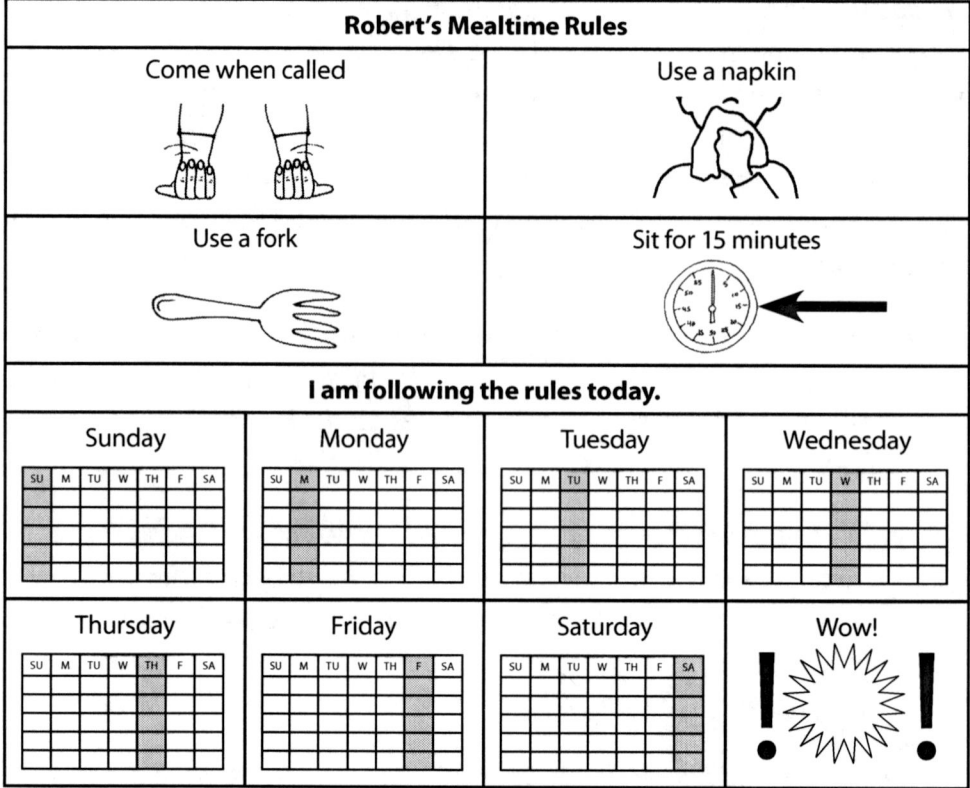

⚙ Tool: Wrong Way/Right Way

In some cases, it is appropriate to include the "wrong" behavior, such as picking your nose, in the visual tool. If you decide to include the "wrong way," be sure to cross it out and show the acceptable behavior next to it. See Illustration 7:2. Don't make the mistake of showing only the inappropriate behavior. This does not give any new information; it does not show your child what to do instead.

Illustration 7:2	
WRONG WAY	**RIGHT WAY**
Hands in pants	Hands in pockets
Yelling, too loud, hurts ears	Quiet voice

Parent Testimonial:

One of the things we've learned is that Cameron responds well to visual cues or representations of "just right" behavior. There is a "right way" and "wrong way" to respond to just about any situation. We have learned that while it may be obvious to us, it's not obvious to him and simply telling him that something is wrong doesn't mean that he automatically knows the right way.

We place a sheet on our refrigerator of the "right way" and "wrong way" for the most commonly used behaviors. It utilizes the universal "no" symbol over the "wrong way" of doing something on the left with red colored ink and on the right, the "right way" of doing something using green ink. The red and green are also universal symbols of stop and go. An example is a picture of a person yelling next to a picture of a person calmly talking. This has worked for all types of behaviors we may be working on. Warning – they may bring the sheet to you when you yell and point out that you've just done something the "wrong way." Beth Kohler

Isaac, age 15, is included in a traditional high school and eats lunch in the cafeteria with other teens. He discovers that he can make the other students laugh by eating non-edibles. His mother is concerned because Isaac believes he is entertaining his "friends." In my office, Isaac describes the items he eats. We list the items one by one, and they become very explicit new rules for eating.

Isaac's Rules:

I will NOT eat:

1. Salad bowls (styrofoam)
2. Ice cream or sandwich wrappers (foil)
3. Forks (plastic)
4. Coins (metal)
5. Dollar bills (paper)
6. Pre-chewed gum
7. Candy wrappers
8. Rocks
9. Trash

I will eat: Food prepared and served in the cafeteria that is on my tray.

Stephen, age 10, rips the pages from books when he discovers a small tear or imperfection. The replacement behavior and new rule become "fix it." After all, this is what we do with things that are "broken" and in need of repair. His mother goes through all of his books and puts those with tears, torn pages, or other imperfections into a special basket kept out of reach on top of a cupboard. When she has time to help him, she takes a book from the basket, gives Stephen a tape dispenser, and prompts him to tape any torn pages together or repair any small tears with tape. Then the book is returned to his shelf. Stephen is rewarded for looking at books without making any new tears. Should he tear a page, the book is removed and placed in the "fix it" basket.

✻ Tool: Red Words and Green Words

Some youth with autism learn to use foul or inappropriate language. Often they don't know what to say instead, but they quickly learn they can cause an uproar and get significant attention for speaking naughty words – classmates laugh and adults get upset. A list can help contain this problem behavior and demonstrate the new rule.

If this is a problem for your child, list the inappropriate words or phrases your child uses in red marker on a whiteboard or piece of paper. These are the "red words." Then decide the words that are appropriate to say instead. These become the "green words." Green words depend upon the context in which the red words are used. See Illustration 7:3. Every time new red words are discovered, add them to the list, along with the appropriate green words. Now the new rule is "Use green words." Whenever the child uses a red word, remind her to use green words by saying something like, "That's a red word. What green word can you say instead?" Show the child the list. Eventually a token system can be added to reinforce the appropriate behavior. See Chapter 9: Using Secondary Rewards.

Illustration 7:3	
Red Words	**Green Words**
This is #%* stupid.	I don't like this.
You idiot!	I'm mad.
Shut up!!	Please be quiet.
You're a loser.	Good game.

✻ Tools for Out and About

Visual rules for specific circumstances, such as in your vehicle, while shopping, at the park, or visiting others can be a remarkable support when you are trying to teach and reinforce new positive behaviors. If you find yourself repeating the rules multiple times, try visual tools.

My child has chronic problems in the community; I can't take him anywhere. He screams, runs away, and even hits me. What should I do?

The Rule is: Stay with Mom.

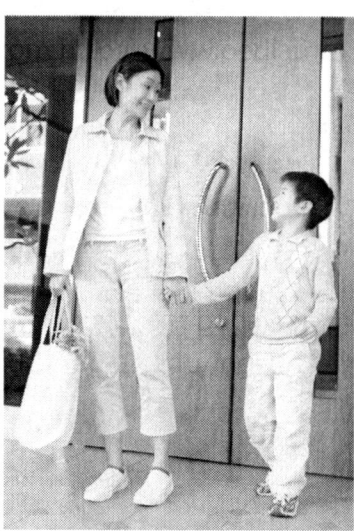

The new rule is "Stay with mom." A photograph of your child standing next to you demonstrates the new rule. Tell your child, "The new rule is: Stay with Mom."

To set your child up for success:

1. Start by exposing your child to places in your community. Begin with short visits that last only a few minutes at most. The length of the activity is a crucial antecedent under your control and one of your best

offensive strategies. Initially, don't expect to shop or accomplish anything except to familiarize your child with the surroundings and teach him the rules.

2. First you might just walk in and out of the store while the child carries the visual tool of rules. Praise him and leave. (It's OK if you have to carry the rules, but keep them front and center so he can see them.)

3. Frequently praise him by saying, "Good staying with Mom."

4. Once successful, on the next trip, you might walk down one aisle, turn around, praise him for following the rules, and leave. If the first trip was not successful, just walk in and out again; then try walking down one aisle the next trip.

5. Make the next trip when the store is not crowded; pick up one item, pay, and leave.

6. Very gradually increase the number of items and time spent in the store until your child is able to follow the rules for 20-30 minutes of shopping; this will take multiple trials.

7. It usually helps to give the child a job while shopping, perhaps searching for items from a photo, putting the items in the cart, counting them as they are put in, or crossing them off the shopping list.

8. Some stores have child-sized shopping carts. These are great for practicing independent shopping.

9. Make sure you have a waiting plan for checkout. Perhaps your child hands you the groceries or helps put them on the belt or scanner.

10. Give a small reward for following the rules. Don't set up the routine of purchasing a treat when you leave the store, because your child will likely expect something the next time. Give the reward in the vehicle at first and eventually not until you arrive at home. After all, he should stay with you for the entire trip.

11. Make a short photo sequence of where you are going "now" and where you are going "next." The sequence might be: home, vehicle, store, home. (See Chapter 6.)

12. Repeat the procedure with different stores and new places (such as a recreation center, restaurant, bank, office, museum).

13. If your child can't tolerate being in a store for more than 5 minutes, then reward after 2 ½ minutes and don't stay any longer than 4 minutes. Set up "practice trials."

14. Expand the store rules if needed, such as in the example below. Review the rules before you get out of your vehicle and praise your child for "good following the store rules" while you are inside the store.
    Store Rules:
    1. Stay with Mom.
    2. Don't cry. Quiet voice.
    3. Listen and do it now.

Rules for good manners and courteous and respectful behavior are "Now and Forever Rules." They usually don't change with the circumstances and are essential social skills. For more information about "Now and Forever Rules," see Chapter 12.

Parent Testimonial:

Cristian is 17 years old and has autism, ADHD and Tourette's. Jordan is 15 years old and has autism, ADHD, and obsessive-compulsive disorders (OCD). Getting the boys ready for school was a challenge when they were younger; mornings were NOT pleasant. We also struggled with bedtime.

Judy helped us to create a rule chart that we posted on all doors – the front door, the bathroom door, and both boys' bedroom doors. The best part of these rules was that they did something magical to my kids – once in writing and posted, they really believed it was a rule and didn't debate with us as much. If they argued or stalled, we told them to look at the chart. When they did it, they earned a token and when they did not, they gave us one back. They used the tokens for extra TV or electronic game time.

We also had a problem with eating at night. They would wait until bedtime and then cry that they were starving; we couldn't calm them down. So we added times and deadlines to the chart. When Jordan asked for a snack at 9 p.m., we told him to go to the chart, which told him no snacks after 8:30, and he would go back to bed. This REALLY worked. All we had to say was, "it's 8:00; you better get your snack before it is too late," and they both did.

D'Anne Ramos

Morning Rules	**Evening Rules**
1. Get up when asked. 2. Get dressed. 3. Wash up and brush your teeth. 4. Fix your hair. 5. Eat breakfast. 6. Get your shoes on. 7. Get your jacket. 8. Get your backpack.	1. Take bath or shower – 8:00. 2. Put dirty clothes in the laundry. 3. Brush your teeth – 9:00. 4. Clean up room – nothing on floor, dishes in kitchen. 5. Turn off TV at bedtime. 6. Snack – 8:30. 7. Cristian bedtime – 9:15. 8. Jordan bedtime – 9:30.

Action Plan for Chapter 7: Teaching New Rules
(Select From the Choices Below)

Rules to Remember:
- ☐ Sometimes the expected behavior is not as obvious to the child as it is to you.
- ☐ Everyone involved must know the new rule(s).

Tools to Use:
- ☐ Wrong Way/Right Way
- ☐ Red Words and Green Words
- ☐ Out and About
- ☐ Other Visual Tool

To Do:
- ☐ Practice Activity 7:1 – Determine the Replacement Behavior
- ☐ The replacement behavior is: _____
- ☐ The new rule is: _____
- ☐ The visual tool is: _____

Practice Activity 7:1 – Possible Answers	
Current Problem Behavior	**Replacement Behavior = New Rule for the child: "The rule is . . ."**
Grabs stuffed animals away from sister.	Trade your stuffed animals with your sister when you want hers.
Pushes brother out of the rocking chair.	Take turns in the rocking chair. Do something else when it is not your turn.
Cries when he loses a card game.	Say "good game."
Cheats so that he can win the game.	Play by the rules.
Tells siblings where to sit at the dinner table.	Let __ and ___ sit where they choose.
Pushes to be first out the door.	Wait your turn. Hands down.
Cries and screams when it's time to get ready for bed.	Follow your schedule with a quiet voice.
Cries and screams when he can't buy something in the store.	Shop from a list with quiet voice.
Won't stay with me in the store.	Stay with me in the store.
Won't keep her seatbelt fastened in the car.	Seatbelt fastened in the car.
Runs out of the classroom when he's upset.	Ask for a break. Stay in the classroom.
Hits his head against the wall when he's frustrated.	Sit and put head down. Squeeze hands.
Takes off her shoes and socks as soon as we are in the car.	Shoes and socks on in the car.
Insists we always eat at Big Boy.	Everyone has a turn to decide where we eat.
Fully tears book pages that have a little tear.	Fix it. Tape the tear and turn the page.
Isn't ready for the bus on time.	Be ready by 7:45.

References and Further Reading

Aspy, R., & Grossman, B. G. (2007). *The Ziggurat model: A framework for designing comprehensive interventions for individuals with high-functioning autism and Asperger Syndrome.* Shawnee Mission, KS: AAPC Publishing.

Green, I. (2003). *Red and green choices: A positive behavior development strategy for students with autism or behavioral predispositions.* Mansfield, OH: Atlas Books.

Horner, R. H., Sugai, G., Todd, A. W., & Lewis-Palmer, T. (2000). Elements of behavior support plans: A technical brief. *Exceptionality, 8*(3), 205-215.

Hudson, J., & Myles, B. S. (2007). *Starting points: The basics of understanding and supporting children and youth with Asperger Syndrome.* Shawnee Mission, KS: AAPC Publishing.

Myles, B. S., Trautman, M. L., & Schelvan, R. L. (2013). *The hidden curriculum for understanding unstated rules in social situations for adolescents and young adults* (2nd ed.). Shawnee Mission, KS: AAPC Publishing.

Chapter 8:

Using Praise and Primary Rewards

L earning new rules and expected behavior is seldom stress-free, so incentives are needed to reinforce the rules and ensure your child masters the new skill(s). Your child requires recognition for his efforts. After all, you are asking him to accomplish tasks that may not be easy for him, and you want him to succeed. Positive reinforcement is an essential tool for your Parenting Toolkit.

What Is Positive Reinforcement?

Positive reinforcement occurs when a reward is provided following a behavior. Simply stated, behavior that is followed by a reward is more likely to occur again.

⚙ Rule: Behavior that is followed by a reward is more likely to occur again.

For example, if your boss informs you that every time you use a new data program correctly, you will receive a $25.00 bonus, you will probably try to figure out the new program and use it often. On the other hand, if your boss warns you that $25.00 will be deducted from your salary every time you fail to use the program correctly, you will also in all probability learn to use the new program. Like most of us, you would want to avoid the "punishment" of money being subtracted from your salary. But in which situation will you likely be happier? I believe that most of us would be happier when we earn the extra bonus rather than losing money.

The same is true for rewarding our children with autism. We want to increase the likelihood that they will do what we ask, not to avoid punishment but to learn a new skill and behavior that they can use for a lifetime, and we want them to feel pleased about their efforts.

Types of Rewards

There are two types of rewards, primary and secondary. *Primary rewards* are naturally reinforcing. They include things like high fives, special privileges, treats, or activities that your child likes. *Secondary rewards* are tokens or tickets. They are not reinforcing alone but must be paired with a primary reward to be reinforcing. When you use a secondary reward, your child accumulates tickets or tokens and exchanges them for preferred activities or privileges. Currency is a secondary reward; it is a means of exchange. By itself it is not reinforcing; it is what you can do with currency that counts (pay your bills, buy groceries, go to the movies, etc.). Once we learn the value of money, it can be a pretty powerful reward!

Examples of Primary Rewards	
Social	Praise, smiles, hugs, tickles, kisses, singing
Material	Art supplies, cars, hair ribbons, flags, action figures, plastic animals
Favorite Food and Drinks	Candies, chips, French fries, cookies, chocolate milk, juice
Favorite Activities	A trip to the pet store, playing in water, swinging, blowing bubbles, shooting baskets, arts and crafts, watching a movie, time on the computer

Social Rewards

Most of us like to be recognized for our efforts, and when we are, we continue to improve and develop our skills.

✿ Rule: Praise builds confidence.

Praise is a wonderful reward and should be a regular part of your vocabulary. It nurtures self-esteem and builds confidence. Some people are meager with encouragement, others don't think it necessary, and yet others are uncomfortable giving it altogether. If you are parenting a child with autism, this is another area where your behavior may need to change. Praise doesn't cost a penny and is readily available and easy to use. Your child's actions mean something, and if you are trying to teach "right from wrong" or "good from bad," the best way to start is to tell her what she is doing right – not what she is doing wrong. She needs your attention for the good things!

✿ Rule: Give attention for positive behavior.

Sometimes as parents we ignore our children when they are playing quietly, eating the way they are supposed to, or simply not bothering us. Then when a child starts to do something we don't like, we criticize. We might say, "Stop fighting," "don't eat with your fingers," or "please be quiet." Perhaps we're in the store and don't say much while the child is behaving, but as soon as he misbehaves, we scold him. Then he has a tantrum, and we tell him that if he can calm down, we'll buy him a treat. The child is getting all of our attention for misbehaving, and he is not learning acceptable store behavior.

✿ Rule: Use more encouragement than criticism.

Search the Internet for the ideal praise-to-criticism ratio, and you will discover answers that vary from 4:1 to 5:1, 6:1, and even 10:1. Regardless of the ideal, it is important to remember that you must be positive more than you are negative. Every time you criticize or reprimand your child, start searching for the next opportunity to encourage him.

When we praise appropriately, we tell our children exactly what they did right. Remember when we identified the replacement behavior and new rule in Chapter 7? Well, this is the behavior that you acknowledge. This rule is what you want your child to master and sustain over time. Therefore, you must let him know when he is making good effort, preferably with a smile and some enthusiasm.

✔ To Do: Practice praising and giving encouragement.

If praise is not part of your everyday vocabulary, the simplest way to begin with young children is to smile and say what you see, "You did it." "You shared your blocks with Sam." "You ate your cereal by yourself." Pairing other social rewards, such as hugs or tickles, with praise can also let your child know you recognize his efforts. Try not to say "good boy" or "good girl." These words don't tell your child what he or she did right. However, sometimes the word "good" followed by the word or words that describe the behavior is initially used with children who have severe language deficits, such as "good__ sitting, listening, dressing, quiet, looking, playing, waiting." As the child's understanding of language increases, use more words.

My child doesn't smile when I praise him. I don't think he really understands what I say and I don't think he cares one way or the other. What should I do?

One of the biggest challenges when parenting a child with limited language is discerning what the child comprehends. Assume he understands more than you think he does. One point to remember is that many children with autism don't react to encouragement in the same way that a typical child does, such as with a smile. In fact, some children with autism get upset when they are praised (most likely because it comes as a surprise and they cannot predict it). But you can assume competence and presume your child understands much of what you say, even if she doesn't speak using as many words as you do or doesn't react in the way you expect. Talk to her as though she does understand – she needs your encouragement and support.

⚙ Rule: Be specific with your praise.

The word choice for praising older children depends upon their cognitive and language abilities, but in most cases you can speak freely. You have an important message to convey, so be as specific as you can. When you feel good about what your child does, say so. If you believe your child comprehends more complicated speech, use entire sentences such as …

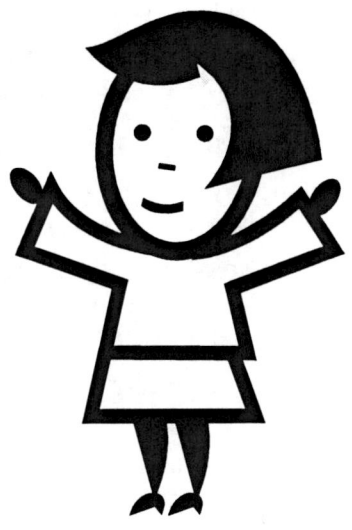

- "Good work getting dressed on time this morning; I really appreciate it."

- "Thanks for helping clear the table. You did a thorough job."

- "Hey, you're doing a great job staying with me in the store; let's stop for ice cream on the way home."

- "Look at Mandy's face. She's smiling because you gave her some of your candy."

- "I like how you waited patiently for me to help you."

- "You must have worked really hard."

- "I like how you keep trying the spelling words, even as they get harder."

⚙ Rule: Praise effort, not just success.

Encourage your child's efforts. When he attempts to do what you ask, follow up with words of support. More words of support that you may want to commit to memory are shown in Illustration 8:1.

Illustration 8:1 Words of Encouragement			
Awesome!	Give me five!	Yes! You did it!	You've got it!
Terrific!	Good try!	Fantastic!	Excellent!
You're trying hard!	Good for you!	I like the way you__	Great effort!

Being Smart vs. Making an Effort

Some children have difficulty admitting that a task is too hard for them, especially if they are told frequently that they are smart. After all, "smart" kids should know how to do everything and don't want to be seen making a mistake. Smart kids are very concerned about making mistakes; they don't want to look "stupid." Be careful if you frequently tell your child she is smart; she may become guarded in the face of challenges and avoid demanding tasks. Instead acknowledge her efforts.

Concerns About Rewards

Many parents express concern about using rewards. They equate rewards with bribes and believe children should be able to act appropriately without a reward. All of us are rewarded for our efforts in our occupations; we are paid a wage, and, if fortunate, receive some retirement and health benefits as well. When we do an exceptional job, we might even receive a bonus. Right now the "job" for your child with autism is to learn appropriate behavior and skills that will lead to being a contributing member of the community, not an easy task.

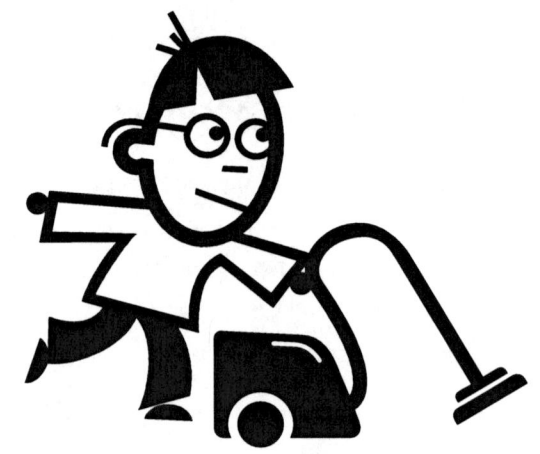

When your child cleans up the toys and you say, "That was a lot of work picking up those toys; you worked really hard. Let's go to the park," you are using a reward. When you show your child the reward she is working for ahead of time, such as a photo of the park, you are using *planned reinforcement*, just like we are usually paid in our jobs, according to a preset plan or contract.

Is It Worth It?

All of us are busy, and parenting a child with autism (or any special needs) is challenging, so there are lots of questions and some anxiety about "Is it worth it?" It takes extra effort to find reinforcers, make charts, keep track of behaviors, administer rewards, and follow through. No one can predict the future, and all children with autism are different, but I can relate numerous stories where incentives helped children learn new skills. Remember, the ultimate reward for you as a parent is to see your child's appropriate behaviors and skills increase. What a great accomplishment. So, "Yes! It is worth it!"

From Now to Eternity

Another parental concern is that once they start, parents will have to use rewards forever. True, we expect to be paid for at least as long as we are doing the work, but often our job responsibilities change and we still receive the same wage (or maybe an increase), and if we take on more responsibilities, sometimes we get a raise or maybe more privileges. The same is true for our children. As their behavior improves, so should their privileges. Your expectations should rise, and so should their responsibilities. Therefore, the reward system you use today will change as your child grows, makes progress, and learns new skills.

Think about potty training. Perhaps you used a small treat to encourage your child to urinate in the toilet. As he learned this skill, the next step was to stay dry, so now he received the treat for staying dry, not for urinating in the toilet. Once he was independent, you no longer needed treats at all, but moved on to teaching another life skill.

"Fair" Does Not Mean "Equal"

Rewarding a child with autism for new behavior raises concerns of favoritism and jealousy from siblings. But remember that every individual has different needs – we all have new skills or behaviors to learn so that we can work towards our maximum potential. Why not reward siblings for their efforts at learning the tasks they need to accomplish? Perhaps you want them to take on more responsibility for taking care of their toys or rooms or some help in the yard or in the kitchen. Perhaps you want them to be kinder, cooperate with each other, and complete a task without arguing. Perhaps their reading or math skills need more work. There are many ideas that you can talk over with them. Just remember, fair does not mean equal.

Now that you are (hopefully!) feeling more comfortable with rewards, let's talk about how to use them. Here are the necessary steps.

1. Determine what behavior to reinforce.
2. Decide whether to use a primary or secondary reinforcement system. (For secondary rewards, see Chapter 9.)
3. Design a reward menu for primary rewards.
4. Decide the schedule of the reinforcement.

Creating a Primary Rewards Menu

Rewards are those activities, small snacks, or objects that you know your child especially likes. Remember, social rewards, such as hugs and praise, are reinforcing, too. The rewards you choose should be something that you know your child will work hard to receive and something that you can limit access to. That is, the reward is saved for the new behavior, and the child may not have it at other times during the day.

It's good practice to create a menu of rewards so that your child has a variety of rewards to choose from and you have a variety of rewards to work with. Once you have a list of potential rewards, rate them with 1, 2, or 3 stars to indicate their potential reinforcement value, with a 3-star rating being the highest.

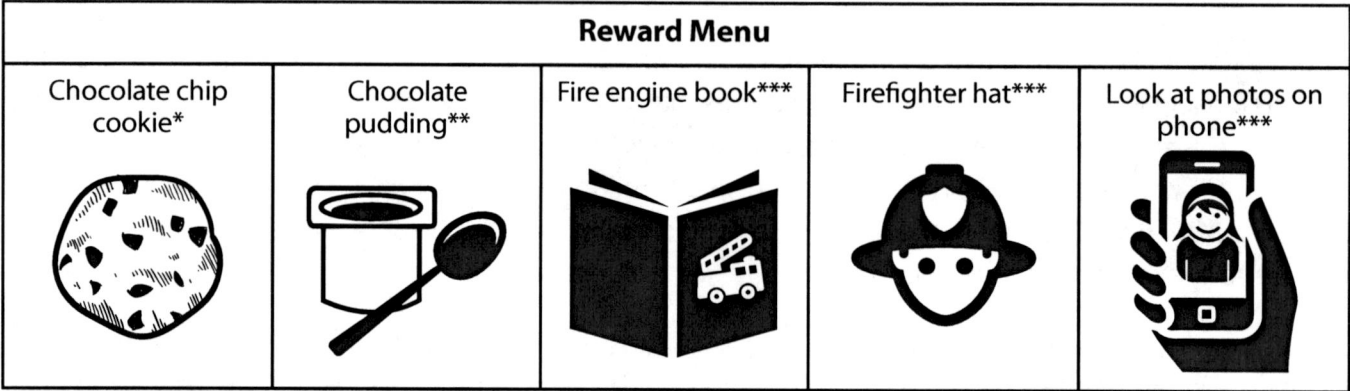

Reward Menu				
Chocolate chip cookie*	Chocolate pudding**	Fire engine book***	Firefighter hat***	Look at photos on phone***

Should I use my child's special interests as rewards?

This is a difficult decision because there is a fine line between a special interest and a fixation or obsession that interferes with daily functioning. Generally, I suggest using special interests, like an interest in the solar system, sports teams, or special characters, as rewards if they are not all-consuming and avoiding obsessions that are already causing significant disruption to family life.

Using obsessions as a reward is often anxiety-provoking and can create meltdowns. Sometimes we think we can control an obsession by using it as a reward. Unfortunately, in my experience this usually fails because the child's obsession intensifies. In other words, we create even more problems as the child becomes more fixated on the obsession and less on the expected behavior. The child's anxiety about NOT earning the reward spirals out of control.

Often, the best approach to managing obsessions and fixations, such as electronics, is to provide them on a predictable time schedule. This is called non-contingent reinforcement. (See Illustration 8:2.) Children don't have to earn non-contingent rewards, but they don't have unlimited access to them either. The only time such a reward is withheld is when the child is demonstrating a severe problem behavior at the time the reward is provided. An example of a non-contingent reward program is the child who receives 30 minutes of screen time every day after school, regardless of his school performance.

✿ Tool: Reward and Activity Surveys

A survey, such as the Reward Survey below and the Activity Survey on page 101 may help you discover rewards that you have not thought of before. Talk with your child's teachers, care providers, and other family members to generate ideas. If you are implementing a brand-new program, such as teaching your child to use the toilet or to wait calmly in line, and you want your child to be highly motivated to succeed, choose a really powerful reward. Include your child in the discussion when possible.

Reward Survey		
Child: _____	**Date:** _____	
Mark the items that you think your child would try hard to earn.		
FOOD		

Candy	❑ M&Ms
	❑ Skittles
	❑ Jelly Beans
	❑ Peppermint
	❑ Chocolate
	  Type_____
	❑ Lollipops
	❑ Candy Kisses
	❑ Smarties
	❑ Fruit Chews
	❑ _____
	❑ _____
		Frozen	❑ Popsicle
			  Flavor_____
			❑ Ice cream
			  Flavor_____
			❑ Frozen yogurt
			  Flavor_____
			❑ _____
			❑ _____	

Cereal	❑ Cheerios
	❑ Trix
	❑ Fruit Loops
	❑ Chex
	❑ _____
	❑ _____
	❑ _____
		Soft	❑ Jello®
			  Flavor_____
			❑ Yogurt
			  Flavor_____
			❑ Applesauce
			❑ Pudding
			  Flavor_____
			❑ Cake
			  Flavor_____
			❑ Doughnuts
			  Type_____
			❑ Frosting
			  Flavor_____
			❑ Cookies
			  Type_____
			❑ _____
			❑ _____	

Fruit	❑ Apples
	❑ Grapes
	❑ Bananas
	❑ Peaches
	❑ Oranges
	❑ Pears
	❑ Raisins
	❑ _____
	❑ _____
		DRINK	❑ Milk
			❑ Chocolate Milk
			❑ Lemonade
			❑ Milkshake
			  Flavor_____
			❑ Juice _____
			❑ Pop
			  Flavor_____
			❑ Kool-Aid®
			❑ Flavor_____
			❑ _____
			❑ _____	

Crunchy	❑ Pretzels ❑ Corn Chips ❑ Crackers ❑ Potato Chips ❑ Doritos ❑ Chex Mix® ❑ Nuts ❑ Popcorn ❑ Caramel Corn ❑ Trail Mix ❑ Granola Bars			

SOCIAL		SENSORY	
	❐ Smiles		❐ Rocking
	❐ Praise		❐ Swinging
	❐ Hugs		❐ Dancing
	❐ Kisses		❐ Spinning
	❐ Tickles		❐ Throwing
	❐ Winks		❐ Dropping
	❐ Clap hands		❐ Twirling
	❐ Rub noses		❐ Pouring
	❐ Whistling		❐ Playing with water
	❐ Singing		❐ Turning water on/off
	❐ Rubbing back		❐ Fans
	❐ Patting		❐ Smelling spices
	❐ Hand shake		❐ Smelling perfume
	❐ High five		❐ Smell other_____
	❐ Piggyback ride		❐ Blowing bubbles
	❐ Chase		❐ Jumping on trampoline
	❐ Peek-a-boo		❐ Playing with zippers
	❐ Hide-and-seek		❐ Playing with flashlight
	❐ Airplane ride		❐ Playing with ribbons/string
	❐ Talk on telephone		❐ Hand lotion
	❐ _____		❐ Balloons
	❐ _____		❐ Mirrors
ART & CRAFTS	❐ Making pictures	**ACTIVITY**	❐ TV show _____
	○ with popcorn		❐ Movie _____
	○ with pasta		❐ Listening to music
	○ with string		❐ Listening to story
	○ with sand		❐ Favorite character _____
	○ other_____		❐ Looking at photos
	❐ Sprinkling glitter		❐ Looking at books
	❐ Drawing/coloring		❐ Playing computer
	○ crayons		❐ Playing electronic game
	○ pencils		❐ Playing ball
	○ markers		❐ Going outside
	○ chalk		❐ Playing with Legos®
	❐ Cutting		❐ Playing with puzzles
	❐ Gluing/pasting		❐ Playing with play dough
	❐ Painting		❐ Bike/wagon ride
	○ Finger painting		❐ Playing with stickers
	○ Pudding		❐ Playing with stamps
	○ Whipped cream		❐ Playing with tops
	○ Soap		

Activity Survey

Child:_____   **Date:**_____

Discuss the activities below with your child and put a check mark next to those that he would like to earn.

	Trip to the park		Extra bedtime story		Swimming
	Eat at a favorite restaurant		See a movie with a friend		Spend the night with a friend
	Overnight with grandparents		Someplace alone with mom		Some place alone with dad
	Later bedtime		Face paint		Jewelry/beads
	Bake		Extra TV program		Trip to garage sale
	Camp in the backyard		Dress up		Special movie
	Go to the library		Rent a movie		Visit the mall
	Shop at the Dollar Store		Order pizza		Trampoline
	Make popcorn		Make a special craft		Visit a friend
	Listen to music		Play a computer game		Visit the zoo
	Treasure box/grab bag		Stickers		Tractor ride
	Car ride		Visit the car wash		Play ball
	Trip to watch airplanes, trains		Choose the menu for a meal		Dance
	Telephone a relative or friend		Ride the escalator in a store		Collect (sports cards, dolls)
	Special snack after school		Special bedtime snack		Art supplies
	Special treat in school lunch		Special breakfast		Books
	Bike ride		Slumber party		Draw/color
	Play outside		Play hide and seek		Swing
	Have a party		Walk		Picnic
	Print page from the Internet				

Setting Your Child up for Success

A sound, well-planned reinforcement program teaches acceptable behavior. When you start a program, thoughtfully consider how you can set it up so that your child will succeed. Here are some rules and tools you can use to help you.

⚙ Rule: Choose a powerful reward for a new program.

Not every behavior change requires a material or activity reward. Your child doesn't need to be rewarded for routine things she already knows how to do, **unless the behavior she already knows how to do is a replacement for a problem behavior** or the **behavior is now expected in new settings**. For example, your child may know how to sit in a chair at the table during meals at home, but when visiting friends or relatives she has trouble sitting and gets out of her seat and crawls under the table. You would not reward her for sitting at the table at home, but you would reward her for sitting at the table while visiting. The point is to make a conscious decision about the reward plan, especially when you are teaching new skills, new rules, or new behaviors.

> *11-year-old John is working on waiting patiently in lines at stores, waiting rooms, or for a meal in a restaurant. Every time he waits without whining, crying, or screaming, he earns a new page from a sports magazine that he likes. He collects the pages in page protectors in a binder and looks at them before bedtime. He also takes the book with him when his family goes to a new restaurant for the first time. This helps him feel more comfortable in the new setting.*

**Add Another Learning Environment
Never Stop Teaching!**

One important point to remember is to never stop teaching. Once a child masters a skill in one environment, move on and teach it in another. Youth with autism often have trouble generalizing what they learn. This means that what they learn in one environment doesn't automatically transfer to another. We have to give them opportunities to learn the new skills in different environments. Therefore, if your child learns to sit at the table in one restaurant (or restaurant chain), move on and practice sitting at the table in another. Use the reward in the new situation. The skill is "sitting at the table," and it will require practice in multiple settings.

It is easy for us to get comfortable and settle into the routine of always eating in the same restaurant because we know our child is comfortable there. But if we want our children to become comfortable eating out alone and with friends when they are adults, we need to start teaching now. Once they have mastered the process, all of you can concentrate on the related social skills that create a successful dining experience, such as greetings, joining in the conversation, or staying on topic.

⚙ To Do: Develop a visual support tool.

A visual support tool demonstrates for your child what to do and describes the consequences for when he does it. In some cases, a photograph of your child engaging in the appropriate behavior is helpful. In others, written words are acceptable. When you change the reward, change the visual tool. If the child has a choice of rewards, illustrate the choices on the tool. Showing your child the reward is acceptable and can be highly motivating.

10-year-old Carmen takes her lunch to school. She and her mother agree that Carmen can put a special fruit snack in her lunchbox if she is ready for school on time. Her mother writes on their whiteboard in the kitchen:

Ready by 7:30 = Treat in lunch box

4-year-old Erica likes to play with rubber snakes. Her mother takes a trip to the Dollar Store and purchases a bag of snakes in preparation for potty training. She plans to give Erica one snake every time she urinates in the potty. At the end of the day, they will count the snakes Erica has earned and start over the next day.

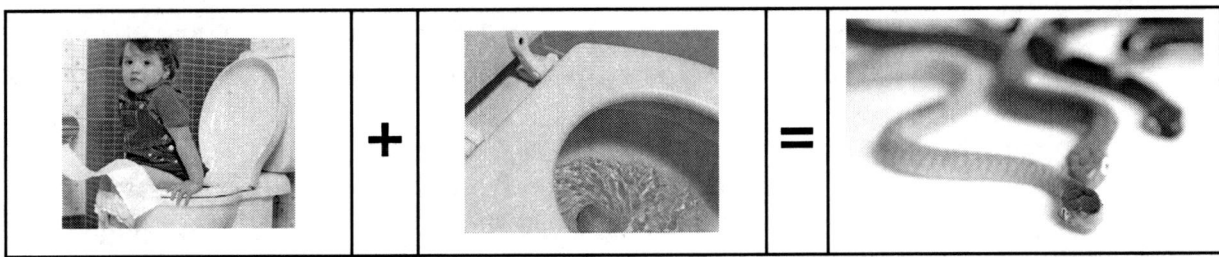

How Much Reward Should I Use?

⚙ **Rule: To reinforce high-frequency new behaviors, use small amounts of the reward.**

High-frequency new behaviors are those behaviors that can occur multiple times a day. Using small amounts of reward for these behaviors encourages the child to continue trying without getting tired of or bored with the reward. This works well for new skills, such as potty training. Remember to pair the reward with praise. Suggested quantities are:

Type of Reward	Amount
Candies and snacks	One or two small pieces
Drink	1 oz.
Television show/movie/computer time	5-10 minutes (use a timer)
Favorite activity (water play, blowing bubbles, music)	5-10 minutes (use a timer)
Story/art project	One story/art project

✿ To Do: Create a reinforcement schedule.

Your next task is to decide which instances of behavior to reward. Do you want to reward the behavior every time it occurs or only sometimes? Types of reward schedules are shown in Illustration 8:2. As illustrated, you have several choices regarding how often and when to administer rewards. Remember your goal is to strengthen the behavior to increase the likelihood that it will occur again in the future. *Continuous reinforcement* is used when you are teaching a new behavior or skill. For example, if you are teaching your child to come to you and you say, *"(Child's name), come here,"* she should be rewarded every time she comes. The reward (e.g., tickles) should be given within 1-3 seconds.

Continuous reinforcement is also used when you want your child to use an alternative behavior instead of a moderate to severe problem behavior (see Chapter 3). When Carmen starts her new morning routine, she receives a special snack in her lunchbox every day she is ready for school on time. After a few weeks of success, she is given a choice of rewards but must be ready on time for two consecutive mornings before she can choose the reward.

Continuous reinforcement requires considerable time and resources and is used for a short period of time only. Once the child has learned the skill or behavior, *intermittent reinforcement* – when behaviors are reinforced only some of the time – can be started using one of the four approaches described in Illustration 8:2. Once a problem resolves, the use of rewards is faded completely. They are gradually discontinued because they are no longer needed. We talk more about this in Chapter 9.

Illustration 8:2 Reinforcement Schedules		
Type	**Definition**	**Examples**
Contingent	Given after an expected behavior occurs and includes the following five schedule types:	
Continuous	Every single time the new behavior occurs	Reward every time shares a toy with a sibling
		Reward every time urinates in the toilet
Intermittent Fixed Interval	After a specific time interval has passed if at least one correct response was made during the time interval	Reward every 5 minutes for working on homework
		Reward every 10 seconds in the parking lot for staying with mom
Intermittent Variable Interval	Behaviors reinforced at unpredictable time intervals	Reward at 10:03, 10:15, 10:20, 10:35 for staying with mom in the store
		Reward at 4:00, 4:30, 5:15, 5:55 for hands to self
Intermittent Fixed Ratio	Reinforce behaviors after a specific number of responses	Reward every 2 pages of completed homework
		Reward every 3 times empties the dishwasher
Intermittent Variable ratio	Reinforces behaviors after unpredictable numbers of responses	Reward sometimes when child follows store rules
		Reward occasionally for following bedtime routine
Noncontingent	Provides rewards on a fixed time or scheduled basis, but children don't have to earn them and they are not withheld (provided the child is not engaging in a problem behavior at the time)	

> **When I want my child to replace a problem behavior with an alternative behavior, how do I decide how long to wait in between giving rewards?**
>
> Look at your frequency count of the behavior problem (see Behavior Logs and Behavior Significance Scale in Chapters 2 and 3, respectively). In general, calculate the average length of time between the problem episodes and divide it in half. If a problem occurs every hour, for example, the reward should be given every ½ hour during which the behavior is not displayed. If a meal lasts 15 minutes and the child gets out of his seat three times, he should be reinforced every 2-½ minutes for sitting in his seat, gradually increasing the length of time when he is successful.

✿ Rule: Reward attempts and approximations.

When using primary rewards in a new behavior support plan, don't expect perfection! Initially praise and reward your child for her attempts and approximations before insisting upon exact fulfillment of your expectations. For example, you and your child are working on transitioning out of the park. In the past you carried her to the car kicking and screaming when it was time to leave, but today she walks to the car crying while holding your hand as you repeat, "Good-bye sand, good-bye swing. See you next time." This is progress, and should be rewarded. On the other hand, if she usually kicks and bites you but today "only" hits you, you would not reward her. Be sure you are only rewarding desired (acceptable) behavior.

✿ Rule: Limit access to the reward.

Finally, the reward you use must be saved for the behavior reinforcement program. For example, your child cannot have free access to television if that is what you are using for the reward.

> *Carlson, age 6, an anxious child with autism who has very limited language, is starting school, and his mother is concerned because he walks with his hand inside his pants touching his genitals. She worries that classmates will tease him and also recognizes that this behavior will not be acceptable as Carlson ages.*
>
> *She makes a new rule, "hands out of pants," and prepares a visual tool. She takes two photographs of Carlson – one with hands in his pants and the other with hands out of pants. She puts the pictures side by side on a chart and places a picture of his favorite snack, pretzels, beneath the photo of hands out.*
>
> *She uses fixed interval reinforcement because Carlson puts his hands inside his pants, on average, every 30 minutes. Dividing 30 minutes in half means he should have the opportunity to earn a reward every 15 minutes. Therefore, she places four tokens on a chart, each designating a 15-minute interval and marked as such with an erasable marker (i.e., 9:00-9:15, 9:15-9:30, 9:30-9:45, and 9:45-10:00). For more about tokens, see Chapter 9.*

Carlson's Chart			
STOP			☺
(hands-out-of-pants icon)	**9:00-9:15** ☹	**9:15-9:30** ☺	(hands icon)
↓	**9:30-9:45** ■	**9:45-10:00** ■	↓
(child washing hands photo)			(pretzels photo)

Initially, Carlson is praised and earns a pretzel every 15-minute time period that he keeps his hands out of his pants. His mom also sets him up to succeed by providing lots of "hands-on" activities, such as playing with play dough, cutting with scissors, and stacking blocks, thus keeping his hands occupied. If he makes a mistake and puts his hands inside his pants, he must wash them at the sink.

Once Carson is successful 80% of the time, he earns the reward after receiving two tokens (30 minutes), then three (45 minutes), and finally all four (1 hour). He has now progressed from getting rewarded every 15 minutes to every hour.

His mom continues to increase expectations, and they start spending more time together in the community where Carlson is also expected to keep his hands out of his pants. Typically, he has something in his pocket to fidget with if he needs it. He visits the neighbors without his mom, so he has a chance to be successful in her absence (she cues her friends to let her know how he does).

Eventually, Carlson is rewarded after an entire day of sustained expected behavior. Now he is ready to start school.

Parent Testimonial:

Often, behavioral goals seem daunting and impossible to achieve. For all involved, it has proven a best practice to build in an incremental reward system to celebrate success along the way. A good example is when we were trying to curb the use of our son's disrespectful language. We made a chart with the words he most often used and their acceptable replacements. On the left was the wrong way to say something using red ink, on the right was the right way to say something in green ink. On the bottom were three squares representing morning, afternoon, and evening. After each part of the day, we placed a candy wrapper (candy was and is still a huge motivator) in the square showing our son's success, and he would get a small piece of candy. If he wasn't successful, the square remained blank for that part of the day, but he could start fresh on the next part of the day. As this method worked, we graduated to a reward system at the end of the day if 2/3 parts of the day were successful.

Beth Kohler

Action Plan for Chapter 8: Using Praise and Primary Rewards
(Select From the Choices Below)

Rules to Remember:
- ☐ Behavior that is followed by a reward is more likely to occur again.
- ☐ Praise builds confidence.
- ☐ Give attention for positive behavior.
- ☐ Use more encouragement than criticism.
- ☐ Be specific with your praise.
- ☐ Praise effort, not just success.
- ☐ Choose a powerful reward for a new program.
- ☐ To reinforce high-frequency new behaviors, use small amounts of the reward.
- ☐ Reward attempts and approximations.
- ☐ Limit access to the reward.

Tools to Use:
- ☐ Reinforcement Survey
- ☐ Activity Survey

To Do:
- ☐ Practice Praise and Giving Encouragement
- ☐ Develop a Visual Support Tool
- ☐ Determine the Reinforcement Schedule
- ☐ The behavior to reward is: _____
- ☐ The reward plan: _____

References and Further Reading

Aspy, R., & Grossman, B. G. (2007). *The Ziggurat model: A framework for designing comprehensive interventions for individuals with high-functioning autism and Asperger Syndrome.* Shawnee Mission, KS: AAPC Publishing.

Downing, J. (2013). Reinforcement. In S. Henry & B. Smith Myles (Eds.), *The comprehensive autism planning system (CAPS) for individuals with autism spectrum disorders and related disabilities: Integrating evidence-based practices throughout the student's day* (2nd ed.). Shawnee Mission, KS: AAPC Publishing.

Swiezy, N. (1999). Changing behavior & teaching new skills. *Disability Solutions, 3*(5-6). Retrieved from www.kennedykrieger.org/patientcare/outpatient-programs/teaching_new_skills

Chapter 9:
Using Secondary Rewards

David refuses to go to school. He dawdles, argues, screams, and even hides. His mother, Shauna, entices him to go to school with the promise that he will get French fries after school. Following a few successful mornings and daily trips for French fries at his favorite fast-food chain, she tries to stop the reward, but David demands French fries anyway. In addition, his resistance to going to school returns. What happened?

1. Shauna did not discover the reason(s) why David didn't want to go to school. So when the reward is removed, the "old" problems are still there.

2. Shauna rewarded the problem behaviors of arguing and screaming even though she thought she was rewarding going to school.

3. Shauna continued a reward that was so powerful that it quickly became part of David's routine, but daily trips for French fries were neither financially sustainable nor manageable in her schedule.

4. Shauna inadvertently set up a new routine (French fries after school) without thinking of the long-term consequences. She forgot to ask herself how likely this new routine would become a problem if it continued (Rule of Five).

5. Shauna failed to clearly connect the expected behavior rules with the reward. As a result, David focused on the French fries and not on what he needed to do to get them.

6. Shauna failed to move to a secondary reward system once she realized how motivating the reward was.

Discontinuing Rewards

One of the dilemmas parents face when using powerful primary rewards (the special privileges, treats, or activities that your child likes) is determining how and when to withdraw them. Some parents stop the reward(s) without warning, believing the child now "knows" what to do and, as a result, doesn't need the reward any more. In cases of skill training, this usually doesn't instigate more problems, because the skill itself is often rewarding, such as riding a bicycle, wearing underwear instead of diapers, or playing a game.

But difficulties occur when parents use rewards to try and change behavior or increase motivation and don't recognize the underlying reasons for the problem. Often, in such cases, a parent assumes the child is choosing bad behavior and withholds the reward to force the child to make a different choice – more appropriate behavior. However, this approach often backfires. When the true reasons for the problems haven't been identified, the child might become more frustrated. That is, not only is he not capable of doing what he is being asked to do, now he has lost his favorite activity(s) as well!

Sometimes parents choose rewards that are not sustainable; for example, they cost too much money, take too much time, or cause other problems in the family. Sometimes the reward isn't a reward at all but a bribe; "Please stop crying and go to school, and I will get you French fries."

Rewards and Rigidity

Youth with autism like predictability, and every now and then routines are established for a child with autism very quickly, such as David. Once such a child starts to earn a reward, he expects to continue receiving it, regardless of his actions. That is, the reward has become part of his rigid routines, even after just a few times of earning the activity.

In similar cases of rigidity, a parent might choose to use a child's fixation as a reward, such as computer time, but the stress of not earning computer time is so great that it causes more problems. If you have a child with strong fixations or one who develops rigid routines quickly, be careful about how you set up the reward program. Be proactive and think of the short- and long-term consequences of your plan, especially whether or not the reward will become a problem (Rule of Five).

In cases of rigidity, secondary rewards become the tools of choice; therefore, don't despair and think that you cannot use incentive programs.

Secondary Rewards

Secondary rewards are paired with a primary reward to be reinforcing. When you use a secondary reward, your child accumulates points, tickets, or tokens and exchanges them for preferred activities or privileges.

What could Shauna – at the beginning of the chapter – have done instead of what she did?

1. David went to school successfully the first day; thus, Shauna knows French fries are a powerful incentive. Even though the reasons why David doesn't want to go to school are unknown, the thought of getting French fries from his favorite restaurant gets him to school, not just once, but for several days in succession.

2. After the initial success on Day 1, Shauna needs a new plan. She could set up a scheduled reinforcement system using secondary rewards. Thus, David continues to earn French fries (or

another reward) when he is ready for school on time without arguing, screaming, and hiding by accumulating tokens or special stickers.

3. David needs a place to put the tokens or stickers and to keep track of how many he earns. He needs a visual tool. Shauna might draw seven boxes on a piece of paper with a marker or on a whiteboard with colored tape, or use a token strip made from a ruler and Velcro. One box is needed for each weekday, one for the number of days needed to earn the reward, and one for the picture of the reward.

Sample Token Strip for David

Mon ★	Tues	Wed ★	Thurs	Fri	2 days =	🍟

4. When Shauna first starts the program, David needs advance preparation; therefore, she shows him the visual tool and explains the plan. The night before Shauna informs David that first he must get ready for school without arguing, screaming, or hiding. When he is ready on time and has met the behavior expectations, he will receive a token (or sticker).

5. Shauna wants David to succeed, so she starts by slowly increasing the expectations. She informs David that when he has two tokens or stickers, he will get French fries after school.

6. Once David has earned two tokens, such as Monday and Wednesday mornings, he receives the French fires after school on Wednesday. They don't have to be consecutive mornings when the new plan begins. The eventual goal is five consecutive mornings getting to school on time without arguing.

7. Once David has earned the reward twice in one week, Shauna can begin to expect that he is capable of earning tokens on three consecutive mornings before earning the reward. For example, if he earns tokens on Monday and Wednesday mornings, followed by Thursday and Friday mornings, the following week he needs tokens for three consecutive mornings in order to earn the reward.

8. If he earns tokens on Monday, Tuesday, and Wednesday mornings, he earns a reward on Wednesday afternoon. If he fails to earn one on Thursday morning, she can remind him that he earns a reward after three mornings and that he might earn tokens on Friday morning and the subsequent Monday and Tuesday mornings. Therefore, he earns a reward on Tuesday. If he finishes that week by earning tokens on Wednesday, Thursday, and Friday mornings, with a reward on Friday afternoon, the expectation increases to four tokens the next week to earn the reward.

9. In this way, Shauna can quickly increase expectations to five days. She must explain the new expectations to David at each stage, show him the changes on the visual tool, and encourage him along the way. David needs to know that his mom recognizes his efforts.

10. Now, to help him be successful, David will also need a visual tool of the morning rules so he knows exactly how to earn a token.

11. A menu of rewards might help to teach flexibility and to let David know he doesn't always have to choose French fries. For example, tokens could be exchanged for other foods or special activities, like a trip to the Dollar Store, play at the park, or visit to a pet shop.

12. Finally, without an understanding of the reasons for David's resistance to going to school, the use of rewards may end up being a temporary solution to the problem. Any skill, knowledge, or social interaction problem must be identified and permanently addressed with a specific plan. Tools to help determine the reason for the problem are presented in Chapters 1-5.

13. Once the underlying reasons have been identified and plans are in place, the expectations might change, but David can continue to earn tokens for meeting them.

> ***How do I decide when my child should earn more tokens before he receives the reward?***
>
> In my experience, it is best to start slowly and gradually increase your expectations. After all, you want your child to be successful. But generally, once the child has earned the reward 2-3 times, it is time to increase your expectations. Don't just stop giving the reward, like Shauna did, but gradually increase the number of tokens needed to earn the reward. This is why it is helpful to have a menu of rewards; some items in the menu might "cost" 1 token, while others cost 3, 4, 5, or even 10 tokens. Then your child can decide how to spend the tokens. Meanwhile, you can expand the program to include new behaviors or skills your child is working on.

Types of Secondary Rewards

There are endless ways to design behavior change and reinforcement programs using secondary rewards. Some ideas of secondary rewards include the following:

Tokens	Tickets	Stickers	Colored dots	Marbles
Colored beads	Smiley faces	Checkmarks	Personal initials	Coins
Coupons	Straws	Collector cards	Stars	Colored stones

There is no magic in what you choose, so think about what is easy for you to administer and simple for your child to understand.

A Colorform® stick-on play set, an easy dot-to-dot picture, or a page from a coloring book with a child's favorite character or special interest can be used for children who have such special interests. When using these options, the child puts on a Colorform piece, connects a designated number of dots, or colors a part of the picture when she meets behavior expectations. When the scene or picture is completed she earns a special activity.

✿ Rule: Choose specific behaviors to reward with tokens, points, or other secondary rewards.

The key to using secondary rewards is to make sure that the expected behaviors are specific. Just saying, "use good behavior, no trouble, or no problems" is too vague and doesn't tell the child exactly what he is to do and what he is not to do. Carlson's behavior plan in Chapter 8 and Carlotta's plan below are very specific. Remember, the desired outcome is increased acceptable behavior, not just reduced undesirable behavior. Let's look at more examples of plans that use secondary rewards.

✿ Tool: Point System

Carlotta, age 10, and her mother struggle to get out of the house on time for school and work in the morning. Carlotta has tightly curled long hair that takes extra care and attention. She has strong preferences about how she wants her hair styled every morning. The problem is that Carlotta is extremely hyperactive and easily distracted. She has trouble sustaining attention to tasks. In addition, she frequently growls, whines, argues, and screams, making the morning extremely stressful for everyone. Efforts to get up earlier have failed.

Mother makes a chart that details Carlotta's morning expectations (see Illustration 9:1). During each activity, Carlotta has two specific rules to follow: (1) use a friendly face and voice and (2) follow directions. She earns two points per activity as long as she follows these rules. If she does not follow directions or growls, whines, or screams, she does not earn the points for that expected activity.

Carlotta and her mother total the points on the way out the door, and during the 10-minute ride to school Carlotta receives the amount of game time that she has earned. Mother gives Carlotta the game at the time that she has earned it. For example, if Carlotta has earned 6 minutes of time, she receives the game 4 minutes into the car ride.

	Get Up	Get Dressed	Fix Hair	Put Shoes On	Eat Breakfast	Rules:
Illustration 9:1 **Carlotta's Morning Plan**						
2 points each						1. No screaming, growling, or whining. Use a friendly face and voice. 2. No arguing; listen, and do it now. Follow directions. Reward: 2 minutes of screen time in the car per activity if meets the rules (a total of 10 minutes).

Here is another example of using a point system.

> *Samuel, age 9, earns points at school for using kind words with others. He earns one point each for being friendly and making nice comments to others without growling, banging his head, hitting, pinching, or using bad words. He earns rewards at the end of the day at home as follows:*
>
> *5 points: put together a Lego Star Wars® set or any activity below*
>
> *4 points: play electronic game for 30 minutes or any activity below*
>
> *3 points: watch television show or any activity below*
>
> *2 points: play with Star Wars® toys or any activity below*
>
> *1 point: Play with trains*
>
> *0 points: none of the above; goes to room and plays with cars*

✿ Tool: Reward Card

A reward card describes a specific behavior or skill that the child is working to increase, such as sharing, taking turns, or waiting. It is small and portable, which makes it easy to use in public. Each time the child demonstrates the expected behavior, a hole is punched in the card or small stickers or stars are pasted on. When the card is completed, the child earns a special treat or activity.

Examples of Reward Cards

Sarah's Sharing Card 1. Smile. 2. Stay calm. 3. Make a sharing plan. Take turns or divide up something.				**Walt's Waiting Card** 1. Stay still, quiet, and calm. 2. Think: "It's hard to wait, but I can do it." 3. Make a waiting plan.		
1	2	3	4	1	2	3
5	6	7	🍨	4	5	6

✿ Tool: Allowance

> *Alyson, age 12, is working to earn new clothes. She earns one dollar each day for the following: Get up without arguing, be ready by 6:15 a.m., feed the cat, empty the dishwasher, get the mail, finish homework, use the clothes chute, pick up the bathroom, do a good deed.*

We first met the Ramos family at the end of Chapter 7. As the boys aged, there was increasing conflict about chores and how well they were completed. During one of our meetings, we discussed the need for a chore chart that specifically included what was needed for each chore. So the family went home and developed one. It has gone through several revisions since then, but their chart is an excellent example of what can happen with collaborative problem solving.

Family Testimonial:

Cristian: *We have had to do weekly chores since we were 5 years old to earn an allowance. We used to have a list that was posted on our bedroom doors of what we had to do to earn our allowance (see Chapter 7). We each got $1 times our grade; for instance, Jordan could earn $5.00 when he was in fifth grade. I had to do at least three extra things to get the extra money since I am three years older. If I didn't, I got the same as my brother.*

My mother always nagged us to do stuff. She complained that we didn't do the chores well enough and that she had to do them over. We were both upset and talked to Judy about it. She suggested we come up with a new chore chart that was more like a job contract. We sat down with our parents and separated each chore/job and wrote out the expectations for it to be done well, how often it would be done each week (some chores, like unloading the dishwasher, get done several times a week), and how much we thought it was worth.

Jordan: *I feel like I had some say about how much chores were worth and thinking up things we could do to help our mom. It feels like a contract, because my brother doesn't always do as much as I, and there were a lot of arguments about who did what. With the chore chart, there is no more arguing, and my mom checks what we did and pays us every Sunday. I have asked to have things added that I think I should be paid for as I have gotten older. Plus, my brother got a real job and hardly does any chores at home, so I asked for a raise and got one. I am very driven by money and I like things in writing, so this works great for me. I think it is fair, too.*

Cristian: *We have been using this chore contract for three years, and it works great. We have rules to follow and some things that we just have to do but don't get paid for. It is up to us to decide how much we do and how much we earn. We have even negotiated with each other to trade some chores that are worth a lot of money and take turns.*

Our mom says it is teaching us life skills, but we both like earning money and being allowed to spend it as we wish, or save for something special. We have shared this chore chart with lots of our friends because it really works!

Mother: *The chore chart works because the boys choose what they want to do and how much money they want to make, but it takes time to work. Give it about a month, and start when the kids are young, like 5 and stop buying them any treats so they have a need for money. When we first started using it, we "wrote it" all together in a family meeting. Then I wrote job descriptions for each job. It is posted on the refrigerator each Monday, and they check jobs off all week.*

I expect at least four things to be done, and they each have to pick a bathroom. Jordan does all he can during the week so he doesn't have to do much on the weekends. Cris usually does everything on Sunday afternoons to catch up, but after a couple months of seeing Jordan doing all the easy stuff, Cris started doing a few things during the week, too. It became a competition.

Later, I added that any chore not completed by the end of the week would be deducted equally from each allowance after one "pass" each month; one week I would do the rest, the next week they paid me if I had to. That is how Jordan got a raise early on, because he did some of Cris's chores, too.

Jordan is the driving force behind the chore chart. He is very motivated by his allowance and willing to work for it. He likes it because he can choose what he wants to do to maximize his allowance, and Jordan earning more money than him motivates Cristian. Cristian only cares when he needs money, so as a team it works every single week. I never have to nag about chores getting done.

It taught them to be responsible and work together, which is hard for brothers to do. I think it helped Jordan feel as if he had some power in the decision-making process. By establishing allowance, as a parent, you have to make them pay for their treats and save for things. I haven't paid for a toy or video game other than for birthdays and holidays in years! Both of my kids are very responsible, good problem solvers, and very good money managers, partly because of this chore chart and how young we started using it.

We have tweaked it as they have gotten older. For example, I added helping with our catering business and yard work, such as mowing the lawn. Jordan has to take care of the dog and clean up after him. Now that Cris is working, he still has to do basic chores, but I only give him money if it is above and beyond or he needs money and is willing to do more. Jordan earns $10-15 a week since he does most of the chores now and still wants to earn an allowance.

As long as the motivation is there, I will keep doing it. I know it seems like everything revolves around money at my house, but the boys both have bank accounts. They pay for gifts for their father and me and each other as well as social activities such as movies or eating out with friends. It really does work if you are consistent.

Cristian, Jordan, and D'Anne Ramos

The Ramos' Chore Chart	
Chores for Free	**RULES**
Clean rooms daily	All chores done by Sunday evening
Change bedding weekly	Allowance is paid on Sunday
Put away clothes	Must be signed as chores completed
Do homework	Maximum to earn is $8 per week
Get ready for day and bed	No fighting over chores
No dishes in room	Rotate every other week – you have the right to decline
No lying	
Hang up coats	No nagging
Get backpacks ready	

Jobs					
Vacuum: 2 times/week How: living room, bedrooms, front hallway	☐	☐			0.50 value/day
Shake rugs: 1 time/week (on weekend) How: bathrooms, kitchen – both doors	☐				0.50 value
Dehair couch & chair: 1 time/week How: Use lint brush roller on arm rests, back, and sides	☐				0.25 value
Empty dishwasher: 7 times/week How: Put all away clean in correct places	☐ ☐	☐ ☐	☐ ☐	☐	0.50 value/day
Load dishwasher: 7 times/week How: all dishes in sink, on counter and stove	☐ ☐	☐ ☐	☐ ☐	☐	0.50 value/day
Empty all trash cans: 3 times/week How: bedrooms, both bathrooms, kitchen; take all outside to dumpster, replace all bags	☐	☐	☐		0.50 value/day
Trash – Tues night: 1 time/week How: take all trash from house to the trash can outside, bring can back to garage Wed	☐				0.50 value
Recycling: 2 times/week (once on weekend) How: take bin into garage, on Tues night take to curb, bring can back to garage Wed	☐	☐			0.50 value/day
Clean small bathroom: 1 time/week on weekend How: use spray and wipe down toilet (inside, back, down the sides), clean both mirrors, use spray and wipe sink and handles and behind sink	☐				$1.50 value
Clean big bathroom: 1 time/week on weekend How: Use spray to wipe down toilet (inside, back, down the sides), use spray and wipe sink and handles and behind sink, use spray and wipe bathtub and sides and rinse out shampoo holder, spray walls with bleach and corners, clean all 4 mirrors and shelf over toilet, use wipe to clean out toothpaste drawer and straighten, use wipe to clean counter and move all, clean cup and replace	☐				$2.50 value
Straighten shoes: 1 time/week on weekend How: put extra shoes in each person's room, vacuum under shoe area	☐				0.25 value
Clean TVs: 1 time/week on weekend How: use glass cleaner to wash all TVs in living room, bedrooms, kitchen	☐				0.25 value
Dusting: 1 time/week on weekend How: every surface in living room, bedrooms – move and replace stuff	☐				0.50 value
Clean TV trays: 1 time/week on weekend How: with wipes	☐				0.25 value
Clean kitchen table & chairs: 1 time/week on weekend How: with wipes, put away stuff on chairs	☐				0.50 value
Clean computer station: 1 time/week on weekend How: with wipes (not screen), printer	☐				0.50 value
Fold laundry: 7 times/week How: sort and fold and put on Mom's bed	☐ ☐	☐ ☐	☐ ☐	☐	0.50 value/day
Bring in groceries: 1 time/week How: carry in and help put all away	☐				0.50 value
Sweep: 5 times/week How: kitchen – pick up rugs, move chairs, and get under counters	☐ ☐	☐ ☐	☐		0.50 value/day
Sweep and dust: 1 times/week on weekend How: use cloth on broom in bedrooms, hallway, and living room, moving all rugs, and under beds	☐				0.50 value
Do what you are asked the first time 7 times/week	☐ ☐	☐ ☐	☐ ☐	☐	0.25 value/day

---

📋 **Action Plan for Chapter 9: Using Secondary Rewards**
(Select From the Choices Below)

⚙️ **Rules to Remember:**
- ☐ Choose specific behaviors to reward with tokens, points or other secondary rewards.

✳️ **Tools to Use:**
- ☐ Tokens
- ☐ Points
- ☐ Reward card
- ☐ Contract
- ☐ Allowance
- ☐ Other

✅ **To Do:**
- ☐ The behavior to reward is: _____
- ☐ The reward plan: _____

References and Further Reading

Aspy, R., & Grossman, B. G. (2007). *The Ziggurat model: A framework for designing comprehensive interventions for individuals with high-functioning autism and Asperger Syndrome.* Shawnee Mission, KS: AAPC Publishing.

Downing, J. (2013). Reinforcement. In S. Henry & B. Smith Myles (Eds.), *The comprehensive autism planning system (CAPS) for individuals with autism spectrum disorders and related disabilities: Integrating evidence-based practices throughout the student's day* (2nd ed.). Shawnee Mission, KS: AAPC Publishing.

Charlop-Christy, M. H., & Haymes, L. K. (1998). Using objects of obsession as token reinforcers for children with autism. *Journal of Autism and Developmental Disorders, 28*(3), 189-198.

Matson, J. L., & Boisjoli, J. A. (2009). The token economy for children with intellectual disability and/or autism: A review. *Research in Developmental Disabilities, 30*(2), 240-248.

Chapter 10:
Building Flexibility

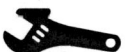

A man once told me that one of his personal rules for functioning was that he had to go in and out of a building the same way – even years later when he returned to that same building, he had to "retrace the trail." This rule helped him manage his day by making one circumstance predictable.

We have spent a great deal of time in this book discussing the fact that most youth with autism like predictability and knowing what is going to happen. This is one of the most important, if not the most important, rules for you to remember.

One evening I found the following message in my email inbox from Sally, age 17:

> *Judy,*
>
> *I just had the worst day ever today. It all started this morning when I tried to put a regular pop in my bag. My mom told me no. Then I got mad. When I was at school, in Computers (the class I struggle with the most), my aide told me to write every word the teacher said in my notes, but I refused to. So I argued with her. Then I got a lunch detention. When I got to the Transition Center, I sassed back to my teachers because they assigned me a different work site. I had to ride the bus home, but I refused to obey. The assistant principal told me to change my attitude and go to work or else lose my summer job and the privilege of being in the work-based learning program. I had the worst day ever, and my lunch detention lasts four days. It is actually called ISS (in-school suspension) where you stay all day.*
>
> *Sally*

What went wrong for Sally?

1. Her mother told her that she could not take a "regular pop" (sweetened, carbonated soft drink) to school; Sally does not know specifically "when" and "how often" she can have one.

2. Her aide told her to write "every word." Sally took this literally – that she had to remember and write every word the teacher said.

3. She was assigned to a different work site without warning, which meant riding the bus home, which she does not like (because of the noise, required social interaction, and delay in getting home).

Managing the Unexpected

All of us have routines; perhaps we sit at the same place at the breakfast table or in a meeting room. Perhaps we drive to and from work using the same route or sit in a preferred chair to watch television. This is normal. It is also normal that most of us adapt to life's daily surprises without too much difficulty. We learn to expect disruptions in our day and manage them to the best of our abilities. We learn to choose to wait or exit the highway if we see construction ahead, go to a different gas station if the one we usually use is busy, select a different book from the library if the one we want is checked out, or stop at the pharmacy on our way home after our spouse calls and says our child's prescription is ready. Maybe we make a mental note for "next time" and take a different route to work to avoid the construction, buy gas earlier in the day, or put the book we want on hold at the library. Such flexibility is typical, and we don't think much about it. Certainly, most of us don't have a meltdown when someone else is "sitting in our chair" or asks us to help with a task.

⚙ **Rule: Multiple unanticipated events can create a crisis for the child with autism.**

For children with autism, who rely on routine and predictability to manage the day, these same unexpected events can precipitate a personal crisis, just as it did for Sally. The underlying reason for the problem is that the child typically has specific expectations for an anticipated event. For example, he expects his teacher to be in the classroom, his buddy to be at the bus stop, frosted cupcakes with sprinkles at a birthday party, or an endless number of other possibilities. But when something unexpected happens, such as a substitute teacher, his buddy is absent, the cupcakes are decorated with jelly beans, the child might become anxious, upset, or maybe more rigid. When there are multiple unpredictable experiences in the course of a day, such as those that happened to Sally, stress builds, and a crisis may be imminent.

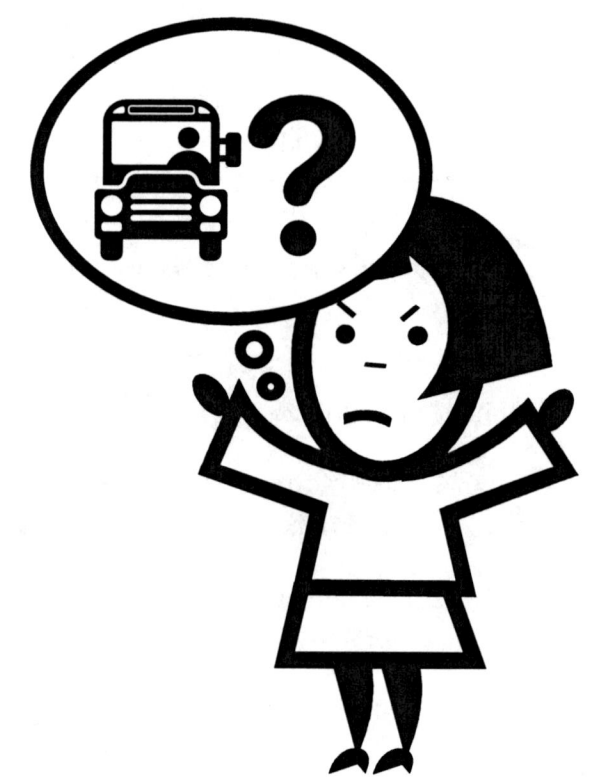

This experience is illustrated in Illustration 10:1. The first event occurs, such as the school bus is late, and the child may become worried. If he does not manage this stress, and another unpredictable event occurs (new bus driver), his stress level will likely increase. If stressful events continue throughout the day, their cumulative effect is likely to cause a crisis for the child resulting in loss of control of his emotions, and perhaps his behavior.

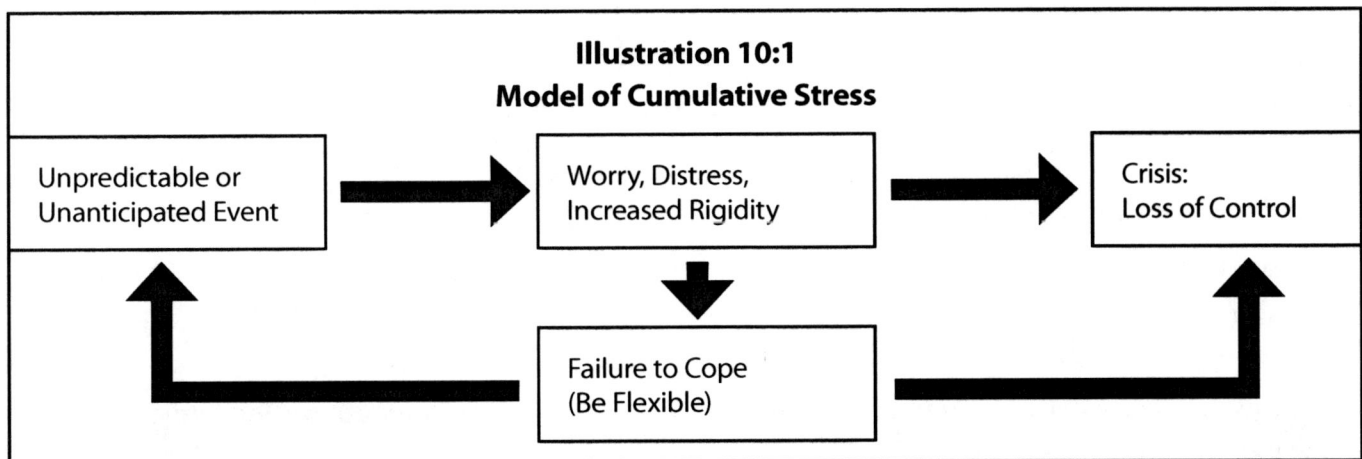

Illustration 10:1
Model of Cumulative Stress

We must teach the tools and skills that our children need to deal with life's surprises and reduce the potential for cumulative stress. However, children also have to learn to recognize, and manage, stress and anxiety when unexpected events occur. Avoidance is not the answer; avoidance simply increases rigidity and reinforces fear of unpredictability and the unknown. There are several critical tools for your toolkit that you can use to help teach your child to be more flexible. In fact, these are tools that you will eventually teach your child to use.

Preparation (Priming)

When introducing your child to anything new, advance preparation is often the key to success. Preparation is the tool used to describe for your child what you expect will happen, how it will happen, and when it will happen. It is just as important as bathing, choosing clothes, or any of the other "get-ready" activities you do before you leave the house. Preparation can be done with an explanation, schedule, visual tool, or a story. The purpose is to give the child as much information as possible in advance in order to minimize the surprises. There will be enough of those anyway, but your goal is to reduce the overall collective stress.

🛠 **Rule: Reducing the total number of unexpected events in a day helps to reduce cumulative stress.**

To prepare, your goal is to describe:

- What's now?
- What's next?
- What if?

For some children, this preparation – also called "priming" (as in priming the pump) – can occur right before an activity, for others it can occur a few hours in advance of the activity, and for yet others, days or even weeks of preparation are needed. This is one of those areas where children with autism vary considerably. It depends upon how often your child is exposed to new experiences, how comfortable she is with change, the communication systems you use, and the level of cumulative stress. If your child is one who asks repeated questions about new events, you likely need to use these tools and prepare her well in advance. When she has the answers to her questions, her repeated questioning will likely diminish, and so will your frustration!

Illustration 10:2
Getting Ready for a Party

You plan to take your child to a family birthday celebration at a restaurant next Sunday. You will need to think about the following:

1. Has he been to the restaurant before? If not, and it is in your community, can you take him to visit and check it out ahead of time? If that isn't feasible, are there photos of the restaurant, for example, on the Internet that he can look at?

2. How will you get there? If your child is someone who likes maps, print out the location and highlight the route.

3. Who will be there? Whose birthday is it? You may need to show him a photo.

4. What is the schedule of events? Ask the host/hostess if you don't know.

5. Will you have to wait or do you have a reservation? What is his waiting plan? (The planned schedule of activities he will do if waiting becomes necessary.)

6. Will you sit in the main dining room or have a private room?

7. Will you order off the menu or will it be buffet style?

8. Check the menu; is there something he will eat?

9. Can you bring alternate food choices if not?

10. Will there be birthday cake and ice cream?

11. Will you bring a gift? Will there be party favors or party bags for the guests?

12. Will he take some tools for interacting with others after the meal is finished (card game, markers and paper)?

13. What is the plan if he becomes overwhelmed or distressed?

Preparation also includes predicting the situations that might go wrong and how they might be managed. The purpose of predicting possible problems is to solve them ahead of time. What if your child doesn't like the ice cream or cake? What if he spills on his shirt or the floor? What if the room is too loud or crowded? What if …? Remember, just because your child knows what to do if he spills on his shirt at home, it does not mean he knows what to do in a party at a restaurant.

All of this advance preparation may seem like a lot of work, but it will be worth it if it makes the entire experience more pleasant for everyone, including your child. He will likely be more eager to participate the next time, and better yet, friends and family members will be more willing to include him, even in your absence. Remember, one of your jobs as a parent of a child with autism is to prepare him for social events in the future.

Sometimes parents question whether all of this preparation is necessary for a child with no or very limited language skills. My answer is, "Absolutely!" It is my experience that receptive language skills are often much higher than a child's expressive skills, so the child will likely understand most everything you say. Keep it simple if you need to, and provide visual tools to help explain what is going to happen. Preparation helps all of us cope with stress, including the child with limited skills. Remember that one of your goals is to help your child be as independent as he can be.

✿ Tool: Getting Ready

The Getting Ready tool in Illustration 10:3 will help you review new situations with your child and give your child a place to check and recheck the information. Start a notebook of completed tools, placing them in sheet protectors. Some youth will be able to write in the information that you provide; in other cases, you will need to write or illustrate it for them. As you find situations repeat, just pull out the paper and make any needed modifications. Write comments or reminders for "next time" on the bottom. Eventually, the goal is for the child to independently research what he needs to know and prepare on his own before a given situation or event.

Illustration 10:3 **Getting Ready for _____**	
1. Where am I going? 2. When am I going? 3. Why am I going? 4. How will I get there? 5. What route will I take? 6. Who will be there? 7. Will there be anyone I know? 8. What will we do? 9. What is the schedule? 10. Will I have to eat anything?	11. Will I get to choose my own food? 12. Will I have to drink anything? 13. Will I get to choose my own drink? 14. What is my waiting plan? 15. What is my calming plan? 16. Will there be any unusual sounds or smells? 17. What else do I need to know? 18. What if …? Comments and Thoughts for Next Time:

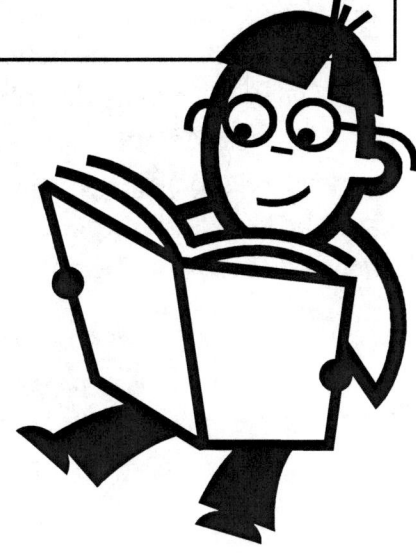

I don't have time for all of this planning and preparation; it's just not my style. I usually don't even decide where we are going until the day before. Sometimes my child does OK, at least for a while, and then we just leave when he has a meltdown.

You have to decide how you can be part of the solution, not part of the problem. Granted, surprises happen to all of us and we decide to do things at the last minute. But that doesn't mean that your child can just "go with the flow." You have to teach him how.

This is what preparation is all about – the more you do it, the less you will have to do in the future, because either the child will be able to do it on her own or the situation will be so familiar that you don't need to. This won't happen unless you give her opportunities to practice and give her the tools to be successful. Unless there is a very compelling reason, staying at home is not an option (see Chapter 12).

Why take a "wait and see" attitude towards meltdowns when you can make a plan that might prevent them in the first place? While meltdowns may not be a big deal to you or your child at this age – they can be a issue for others around you, and certainly are not behaviors we want to encourage. Remember the Rule of Five.

When you truly don't have time to prepare, give the job to someone else, a sibling, grandparent, or spouse, and if all else fails, do it on the way to the event.

⚙ Rule: Getting ready for new experiences is the key to success.

Advance planning for any situation in which you know your child will be especially anxious or fearful is vital if he is going to learn how to cope. This is especially helpful in situations that are seasonal or tend to repeat, such as a fear of storms or a fear of insects. Getting ready is the key to success. In these situations, you and your child determine the plan together.

Gardner and Jaffe (2006) illustrate one method to help children prepare for stressful situations in their book, *How to Control and React to the Size of Your Emotions – An Interactive Workbook for Parents, Professionals, and Children*. The basic procedure is that the child first identifies the overall emotion, such as fear of storms. Then he describes the size of the emotion (little, medium, big) by its details, and finally develops a specific plan for each one. This approach is successful because ultimately it provides the child with a concrete plan of what to do in each situation. It makes the situation predictable and because he knows his options, stress is reduced and quite frequently, the problem is resolved. Remember, each child's plan will be different because circumstances differ and each child is different.

> *Ben, age 10, has an intense fear of storms. He is vigilant about checking the weather forecast every morning and becomes distressed when dark clouds appear in the sky. He is watchful all day if a storm is predicted and is unable to go to bed at night. After implementing his Storm Plan (Illustration 10:4), his hyper-vigilance subsided, and storms were no longer a source of extreme fear.*

Illustration 10:4
Ben's Storm Plan

Things that make me afraid:		
LITTLE FEAR	MEDIUM FEAR	**BIG FEAR**
Strong wind	**Thunder and lightning**	**Hearing about a tornado on the weather channel**
Dark clouds	**Power failure**	
When the tree outside my bedroom bangs on the window	**Storm warning on television**	**Tornado watch/warning on the television**

What I can do:		
LITTLE FEAR	MEDIUM FEAR	**BIG FEAR**
Go to a safe place inside a building.	**Get my mom or dad.**	**Mute the TV.**
Don't look out the window.	**Get my flashlight.**	**Look at the atlas and find out where the tornado or storm is.**
Think about my favorite things.	**Sleep by the fireplace if it is cold.**	**Go to the basement under the stairs.**
Talk to someone.	**Ride to Tom and Mary's house.**	**Check for windows.**
Close the curtains in my bedroom.		**Play a game.**
Turn on my radio.		

Flexible Thinking

Most children with autism don't do well when others have a different opinion, another way of doing things, or preference other than their own. In fact, they consider any suggestion to consider, and perhaps adopt, another's point of view absurd. Such youth are not being selfish; they simply don't understand that other people may have different ideas and that all opinions have equal merit. Furthermore, like many of the children you have met in this book, they don't appreciate that they should have to consider these other opinions and come to an agreement on a solution that is mutually acceptable.

Consider putting together a multi-piece puzzle. First you might try to fit together two pieces. If you can't find one that fits, you try another. You might start with the edge pieces and work towards the center, or you might start with a corner and fill that in first. If you are working alone, you might ask for help. The point is: There is no one right way to work at it. There are many strategies for putting a puzzle together, and all of them are OK.

⚙ Rule: Flexibility = More than one right way.

One of our goals is to help your child understand these basic tenets of life and learn to handle risks. Your child will become more flexible by understanding that there is more than one way/one answer/one opinion/one direction/one choice. **Telling your child is not enough;** you have to live out loud at the time a problem is happening to you, and show her how you cope by your actions.

✿ Tool: Think out Loud

Your voice is helpful to your child when you are faced with any of the mundane, and typical, problems that happen in the course of the day while you are with your child. Instead of keeping your thoughts to yourself, think out loud.

Declare what is happening such as, "There are too many people in this check-out line; it's taking too long to check out." Then state possible solutions: "It's no big deal. I can handle this; lines 2 and 3 are pretty short. I can move over. Line 2 looks shorter, we'll move there. Then we should get done in time to pick up Sarah from her ballet lesson." When you think out loud, you are identifying for your child:

- What is happening here? What is the problem?
- What else can I do?
- What might happen next?

You are also modeling positive self-talk, another tool that helps all of us cope with stress and anxiety. Positive self-talk builds confidence!

✿ Tool: Model Positive Self-Talk

Self-talk is an essential tool in another area where youth with autism frequently struggle – dealing with mistakes. Most mistakes can be corrected, undone, easily forgotten, or apologized for, so why take them so seriously? But some children are greatly affected by mistakes. Afraid of making one, some youth don't even start an activity. Others are afraid of making the wrong choice and, therefore, don't choose at all. Some youth second-guess decisions and are never sure they have made the right choice. Others have severe emotional reactions after making a mistake (or when someone corrects them or someone else makes a mistake). Often these reactions are related to thoughts of "only one right answer, way, or choice."

Some youth cannot accept responsibility for personal mistakes; they are always someone else's fault: "I was late for school because mom didn't have breakfast ready on time." "You made me do it." "I couldn't clean up because Johnny was bothering me." Self-talk models for your child how to assume responsibility for personal actions and deal with mistakes.

Help your child look at mistakes with humor and grace. Yes, it is disappointing to have to start all over again, get a low grade on a test, fall off a bicycle, spill your juice, but it's really no big deal. Phrases you can use to model self-talk with your child are shown in Illustration 10:5.

Illustration 10:5 Positive Self-Talk		
It's no big deal.	I can handle this.	I'm O.K. Let it go.
No problem.	I'll be fine.	I'll do better next time.
I can do this!	I can try.	It's not so bad.

✹ Tool: Visual Supports

Discussed extensively in previous chapters, and required to build flexibility, are your visual communication tools. Showing your child there are multiple ways to make decisions is critical when teaching flexibility. Remember that visual supports can be pictures, written words, photographs, line drawings, or actual objects.

Miguel, age 6, dictates where his siblings sit at the table. But they want to decide themselves where they sit, so there is a lot of arguing and fighting right before mealtime. Miguel's mother chooses to draw shapes (triangle, circle, square) on plastic placemats because all of her children are quite young. She draws the same shapes on note cards. Each meal the children take turns putting the placemats on the table; then each child draws a card from an envelope and sits where the matching shape is located.

Terry, age 10, has trouble getting started with his morning routine every day. He argues with his parents and doesn't want anyone to tell him what to do. His dad prepares five job cards: put on shoes and socks, eat breakfast, brush teeth, put backpack by the door, and get dressed. He hands the cards to Terry every morning with the directions to complete the jobs in any order.

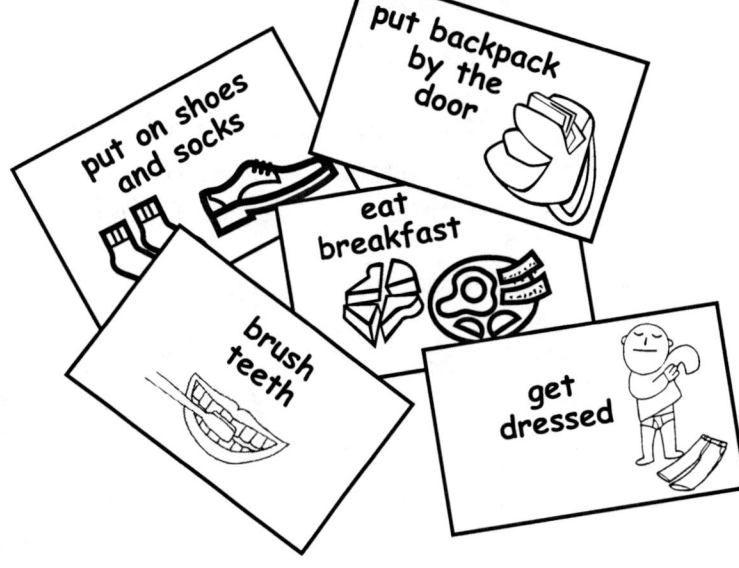

Visual communication helps children to "see" how decisions are made and, ultimately, increases their flexibility and reduces rigid preferences. Over time, when used consistently, visual tools show the child a systematic and different way to make a decision, illustrating there is more than one "right way." Eventually, the tool is no longer needed because the child learns there are multiple ways to make decisions and there is no one right answer, decision, etc. The process becomes the routine, and in due course it is no longer needed.

Visual tools can be used for many daily decisions, such as a child's place in line, turn to do an activity, place to sit, or restaurant to eat at. Letters of the alphabet, numbers, photographs, animal pictures, notes, or any symbol can be used, depending upon the age and functioning level of the child.

> *Eight-year-old Mark insists that his parents drive to school via the same route every day. They decide to show him that there are multiple ways to get to school. They print a map of their neighborhood from the Internet and make several copies. Then they highlight a different route on each map and place them in a large envelope. Each day Mark pulls a map from the envelope. He follows along on the map while his parent drives. Now he is learning all of the different ways he can get to school. There is no one right way!*

❁ Tool: "What If" Situations

Teaching your child to be more flexible requires practice, preferably in situations where both of you are calm and relaxed and know what to expect. To do this, set up "What If" situations and practice with your child exactly what to do. This is especially helpful when your child goes into meltdown mode when his rigid preferences are not met.

"What If" There Is No More?

Perhaps your child has a favorite ice cream flavor and you keep the freezer stocked with that flavor to prevent a meltdown. Although this is an easy solution for now, what happens if you run out, have a power failure so it all melts, or forget to buy some? Let's walk through the steps of how to teach your child what to do when there is no more of his favorite flavor of ice cream.

Guided Practice: No More Chocolate Ice Cream

Sit down with your child and generate a list of all the desserts he likes (flavors of ice cream, types of cookies, cakes, fruits). Pull the items out of the refrigerator or cupboard and show him if needed. Then put them back.

Now have him prioritize the list; what is his top favorite, next favorite, third favorite, etc.? Number them.

1. Now talk about "What If." "What if you go to the freezer for chocolate ice cream and there isn't any, or I tell you there isn't any more?" Actually walk to the freezer, open it, and talk about this. (Don't remove the ice cream.)

2. Now, discuss the choices on the list. "It's no big deal. There are lots of other desserts you like, too. Let's see what we have. Well, strawberry ice cream is on your list as your next favorite. I see we

have both strawberry and vanilla ice cream. Let's look in the pantry. We have chocolate chip cookies and sugar cookies. They are on your list, too. You have lots of choices."

3. "So, if there is no more chocolate ice cream, what could you choose? You like all of these desserts; you have lots of choices." Repeat the choices if necessary.

4. After your child chooses, say something to the effect of: "Good plan. We'll practice it again tomorrow," and let him have some chocolate ice cream if he wants; if he chooses another treat, that is fine, too. Post his list in a prominent place and suggest that he write chocolate ice cream on the shopping list.

5. Practice for a few days in a row; then say, "tomorrow there will be no more chocolate ice cream. We are going to try your new plan."

6. Then do it.

7. Keep practicing in multiple situations (restaurants, friends, and relatives).

8. Repeat the process with "no more" of his first and second choices, then third choice. You want him to see that there isn't just one best choice, often there are lots of choices, and all of them are OK.

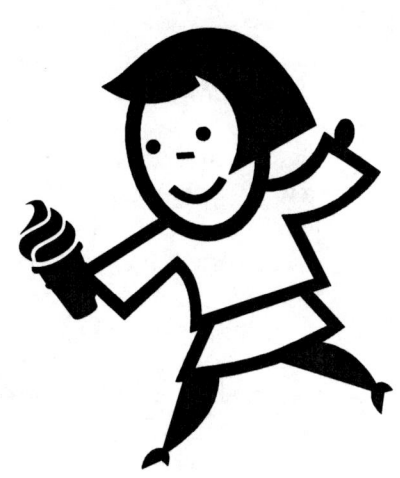

9. Introduce and set up guided practice of "What if" for other rigid expectations one at a time.

There may be a few bumps along the way as you practice the "What if" situations, but the more opportunities your child has to practice being flexible, the greater the likelihood he will become more flexible. "What if" you continue to reinforce his rigid preferences? Then flexibility will likely never happen. The key is to practice in advance!

"What If" There Is a Schedule Change?

Schedules help make life predictable and are important for reducing overall stress. Schedules are an essential tool in your Parenting Toolkit (see Chapter 6), but what if you need to stop at the pharmacy, pick up a gallon of milk, or the gas gauge is running on empty? How can you teach your child to tolerate such changes?

First of all, you must have the schedule firmly and consistently in place, a predictable system for the child to check "what's now and what's next," and one that he can trust to be true. If you change what you do without changing the schedule, your child can't trust your system, so he has to be extra vigilant to make sure you follow it. On the other hand, if you don't use a schedule at all (because it takes too much work, too much time, you forget), then your child is kept in the dark, which may cause even more anxiety.

If your child consistently reacts negatively to changes in routine or changes in plans, schedules are essential for teaching flexibility. Illustration 10:6 lists rules and tools.

Illustration 10:6
Rules and Tools for Changing the Schedule

- Keep a small whiteboard in your vehicle or photographs of the places you frequent. For durability, photos can be laminated or kept in page protectors. Some parents choose to keep photos on smartphones or in a photo album in the glove compartment.

- Write the schedule on the whiteboard or sequence the photos in the order you plan to use them.

- Depending upon the age and functioning level of your child, choose a written or photo list of several activities. You may have to experiment to find out the ideal number of items to include on the schedule at one time. Start with "now and next," or "first, then," showing just two activities. Add more activities as each is finished.

- Start to add activities to the schedule that you know your child likes, such as a stop at the pet store or a walk to the park. Show your child that all changes in the schedule don't have to be "bad." If you are writing on a whiteboard, you can say, "Oops, I forgot to add in pet store. I'll write it here, and we'll go to the pet store first and then we will go home."

- Another way to add in changes is to cross out what you are not going to do and replace it with what you're going to do instead. "It's so nice out today, let's go to the park instead of grocery shopping. We can buy groceries tomorrow." Then cross out grocery shopping and write in park.

- As your child is successful, start to add in activities your child doesn't like. "The gas tank is almost empty; we need to buy gas before we go home. I'll put it on the schedule." Sometimes including a preferred activity after a non-preferred activity is helpful. "I don't feel like cooking tonight; let's go through the drive-through after we buy gas."

A Word of Caution

Be careful about setting up new routines or patterns that are difficult to sustain. For example, if you go to the drive-thru after you buy gas several times, your child will begin to expect to go through the drive-thru after you buy gas every time. The secret is to use the schedule to show what's going to happen next, but don't establish a new routine unless you intend to make it a "now and forever" routine. In other words, the next time you buy gas, just go home afterwards and use the schedule to explain this to your child.

Parent Testimonial:

Next, Now, Finished

Cameron is fully included, and his elementary school utilizes supplemental classroom teachers in addition to the regular teacher for various subjects. This, coupled with specials like media, technology, music, lunch, etc., meant a day full of transitions for a kid who didn't handle transitions well. It wasn't that he wouldn't transition, but he was riddled with anxiety about when the transition was going to occur, where he was going next, and who would be there. The perseveration prohibited him from participating in the current activity – whatever it was. The solution was a "Next, Now, Finished" chart made up of laminated pictures (the more realistic the better) with Velcro® backing placed on his desk to indicate the current activity and what was next. When he was finished with the current activity, he placed the chart in the "finished" pocket, moved the next activity to "now" and placed the "new," next activity in the appropriate spot. This system was so popular with the other kids in his class that they always came over to his desk to see what was next. Eventually, the teacher made a life-sized chart for the entire class to use.

Beth Kohler

Slowly we are filling your Parenting Toolkit with the tools you need to solve problems. What about strategies for those persistent problems that don't seem to change? Complete your Action Plan below, and let's find out what to do in Chapter 11.

Action Plan for Chapter 10: Building Flexibility
(Select From the Choices Below)

Rules to Remember:
- ☐ **Multiple unanticipated events can create a crisis for the child with autism.**
- ☐ **Reducing the total number of unexpected events in a day helps to reduce cumulative stress.**
- ☐ **Getting ready for new experiences is the key to success.**
- ☐ **Flexibility = More than one right way.**

Tools to Use:
- ☐ **Getting Ready**
- ☐ **Think out Loud**
- ☐ **Model Positive Self-Talk**
- ☐ **Visual Supports**
- ☐ **"What If" …**

To Do:
- ☐ **One situation to prepare and plan for is:** _____
- ☐ **The preparation plan is:** _____

References and Further Reading

Baker, J. (2008). *No more meltdowns.* Arlington, TX: Future Horizons.

Dalrymple, N. J. (1995). Environmental supports to develop flexibility and independence. In K. A. Quill (Ed.), *Teaching children with autism: Strategies to enhance communication and socialization* (pp. 243-264). New York, NY: Delmar Publishers, Inc.

Gardner, L., & Jaffe, A. (2006). *How to control and react to the size of your emotions – An interactive workbook for parents, professionals, and children.* Shawnee Mission, KS: AAPC Publishing.

Hodgdon, L. A. (1995). *Visual strategies for improving communication, volume 1: Practical supports for school and home.* Troy, MI: QuirkRoberts Publishing.

Hodgdon, L. A. (1999). *Solving behavior problems in autism: Improving communication with visual strategies.* Troy, MI: QuirkRoberts Publishing.

Koegel, L. K., & LaZebnik, C. (2004). *Overcoming autism: Finding the answers, strategies and hope that can transform a child's life.* New York, NY: Penguin Books.

Moskowitz, L. J., Carr, E. G., & Durand, V. M. (2011). Behavioral intervention for problem behavior in children with Fragile X Syndrome. *American Journal on Intellectual and Developmental Disabilities, 116*(6), 457-478.

Myles, B. S., & Hudson, J. (2007). *Starting points: The basics of understanding and supporting children and youth with Asperger Syndrome.* Shawnee Mission, KS: AAPC Publishing.

Chapter 11:
Changing Routines and Fixations

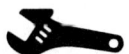

The balance between maintaining predictability and teaching flexibility is tenuous. You have likely heard about children with autism who always have to be first in line; in fact, they may push others away or have a tantrum if they are not first. Some want to ride the same way to school every day or take the same route to the grocery store. Like the children in Chapter 10, these children are striving for predictability – to "know" exactly what's going to happen. They will make up the rules to create predictability if none exist. In their quest to keep things predictable, they develop rigid rules, and these rules often become a problem for everyone. Remember 4-year-old Jack from Chapter 3? Jack's rule was that only he can open or close a door in the house. It's easy to imagine how this rule can be challenging for others in Jack's life.

⚙ Rule: If you don't make up the rule, the child may do it for you.

Frequently, youth develop rigid rules when the real rules in a situation are unclear or unpredictable. Why Jack developed his rigid rule in the first place is difficult to discern, but it is likely because he doesn't know precisely who is going to open the door and enter or leave the house at any given time. The behavior appears arbitrary, and this unpredictability in his busy household is unacceptable to him. He tries hard to execute his rule and when other members of the family violate it (by coming in or going out unexpectedly), he becomes frustrated and angry and tries even harder to enforce his rule, making life exceptionally stressful for everyone.

To solve this problem, Jack needs a "new rule," one that fits the problem situation, yet provides predictability and fits the Rule of Five.

Persistent Problems

When your efforts to improve a situation meet with failure, it is time to decide if a new rule or routine is needed. The following are indications that a problem situation needs **more** structure and predictability:

1. When the problem is constant or happens at the same time almost every day, such as in the morning, after school, or at bedtime.

2. When the problem happens every time the same situation occurs.

3. When the problem is significant (see Chapter 3).

✹ Tool: Come up With a "New Rule"

Generally, new rules for a child with autism are "universal rules" for the rest of us. They are what we would typically do in the given situation. In this case, Jack's "new rule" is that any family member can open or close a door. Although it is quite evident to us that anyone can open a door, it is not obvious to Jack. This is a new rule from Jack's point of view. This brings us to another fact about parenting a child with autism: Often what is obvious to us is not obvious to our child.

✹ Rule: What is seemingly obvious to others is not obvious to some children with autism.

✹ Tool: Change the Routine

Now that we have identified the new rule, there are two goals to achieve. The first is to successfully communicate the new rule to Jack. The second is for Jack to accept the new rule without arguing or fighting. We want Jack to understand that it is OK for anyone to open or close the door. How can we help him? His parents have tried to tell him, and his siblings have even opened/closed the doors in frustration. It is likely family members quietly creep about the house, secretly coming and going, hoping Jack doesn't realize their movements. Unfortunately, this just increases his vigilance.

So what can they do? They need a new routine that replaces their usual behavior habits and one that establishes normalcy to the household. It cannot be "business as usual" for the sake of everyone's sanity.

Photographs are chosen as the way to communicate the new rule to Jack. They are powerful and permanent tools of communication when used consistently. They are stationary, do not disappear like words do, and, most important, they communicate to Jack exactly who is opening the door.

Photos are taken of each family member, and one set is placed in an envelope at each exit. Next, the new routine is established and practiced. The family gathers at the door, and the new rule is explained to Jack: Anyone can open or close the door. Jack is asked to select a photo from the envelope. The person depicted goes first, and opens and closes the door. Everyone cheers. They practice the routine several more times, showing Jack that anyone can open or close the door and it is OK. A reward system is put into place for "following the new rule."

The next time family members get ready to leave the house, their photos are placed in the envelope. If Jack is also leaving, his photo is included. If Jack (or any other family member) is not leaving, his or her photo is left out. One of those leaving the house chooses a photo and that person opens the door.

If Jack protests, he is reminded of the new rule. Eventually, Jack learns that anyone can open or close the door. He relaxes. After a few weeks, photographs are no longer needed, family members come and go as needed, and this very significant problem is resolved.

This plan for Jack emphasizes the importance of communicating in a way the child can understand. What seems an obvious expectation to us may not be so obvious to the child. So one task is to ensure the child truly understands our expectations by making that information as explicit as possible.

This seems like a lot of work and effort. Let's say it takes 15 minutes to print photos and 15 minutes for family members to practice the new routine with Jack. It takes another 1-2 minutes to put the photos in the envelope and go through the new routine every time someone goes in or out of the house. So maybe a 2-hour investment per family member. But think of it this way: How much does it "cost" each family member for Jack to melt down? How much time does it take to let Jack open and close all the doors? The investment of 2 hours seems well worth the alternative costs of letting Jack keep this rigid rule.

Six-year-old James takes aripiprazole, a medicine used to treat mood symptoms. One of its adverse effects is increased appetite. Every day after school James and his mother argue about what snacks he can have and how much he can eat. He wants cookies, chips, and candy. She wants him to eat healthier snacks. He badgers and bullies her into allowing him to eat what he wants. He has a meltdown and becomes aggressive if he doesn't get his way. Often he ends up in his room crying and screaming while his mother is in tears. James' food choices must be closely monitored because he is gaining weight. What can his mother do?

James probably has some idea of the snacks he wants after school, but when he comes home, mom tells him no. Her reaction is unexpected from his point of view (he expects her to agree). Her reaction is also unpredictable – sometimes she says yes and sometimes she says no. So how can she make the situation more predictable?

✿ Tool: Change the Routine

Considering what is reasonable, what fits the Rule of Five, and what adds predictability, what is the "new rule," how is it communicated to James, and what is the new routine?

James' parents decide it is reasonable for him to have one healthy snack (piece of fruit/yogurt/cheese) and not-so-healthy snack (chips/cookie) after school. To make this rule very clear and specific for James (who doesn't read), a red- or green-colored sticker is placed on every snack container. "Unhealthy" snacks receive a red sticker while "healthy" snacks receive a green. When James comes home from school, he is given one red and one green card, and is then directed to "spend" his cards, choosing one snack of each color.

What has happened as a result of this plan? First of all, all the snack choices become predictable for James; they are either red or green. He also has a predictable routine every day, one red and one green card to spend on snacks. He can think about his choices all day if he wants, perhaps deciding in advance what snack he prefers, and he is secure in the knowledge that when he comes home his mother will not say no. Maybe one day he wants pretzels and the next day he wants cookies. Now that the choices and expectations are clear for both of them, they have a much calmer afternoon, with no more arguing or meltdowns over snacks.

Yes, it takes time and effort to place the dots and use the cards, but the benefits are well worth it. Reducing the total number of stressful events in a day helps to reduce cumulative stress, so when you set up a new routine for persistent, predictable problems, you are removing one of the obstacles to a successful day.

> ***Why does she have to use colored dots and cards? Why not just tell him that he can choose one healthy and one unhealthy snack and then follow through?***
>
> James needs reassurance. The colored dots and cards show him exactly what he can eat. He can check and recheck as often as he wants. Remember that visuals are permanent and stationary. They make the choices clear for everyone, a babysitter, grandparent, or anyone else who needs to know and support the new rule.

Power of Choice

There is another influential element in these examples that you may have noticed – the power of choice. Like most of us, youth with autism like to make their own choices, and once they have made a decision (or choice), it is difficult to change. When a parent wants the child to make a different choice, a power struggle occurs. So allowing James to choose his snacks within specific guidelines and then consistently following the guidelines is a win-win. In this case, his mother is effectively setting up a new routine that includes meaningful choices for James, and the power struggle is avoided. Let's look at more examples.

> *Five-year-old Mohammad is in kindergarten. He resists completing any "homework," which typically consists of reading for 10 minutes after school. His mother prefers that he "read" soon after he comes home, but Mohammad wants to play. If his mother allows him to play for a short while, he still argues and yells at her when it is time for homework. She is exhausted and overwhelmed (partly because she is also taking care of a newborn infant), and Mohammad is irritable, angry, and upset. What can she do?*

✿ Tool: Change the Routine

Again, considering what is reasonable, what fits the Rule of Five, what adds predictability and includes choice, what is the "new rule"? How is it communicated to Mohammad and what is the new routine?

Mom prepares four cards for Mohammad, one says, "homework – 10 minutes" and three say, "playtime – 10 minutes." All have picture icons (book or toys) to show Mohammad what homework and playtime mean. Mother explains the new rules and routine to Mohammad. When he comes home from kindergarten, she hands him the four cards. His job is to put the cards on the table in the order he wants to do them. It doesn't matter what order he chooses. Then they set a timer for 10 minutes, and Mohammad proceeds with the first card. When the timer rings, they turn over the first card, set the timer again, and he moves on to the next card. When he is finished with all four cards, he chooses a snack. In addition, he earns a special card for "following the rules" that can be exchanged for special privileges. (For more about rewards, see Chapters 8 and 9.)

It doesn't take Mohammad long to learn the new routine. He likes deciding how to spend his time. Interesting, he usually chooses to complete homework first, thus leaving more time for play (which his mother wanted him to do in the first place!).

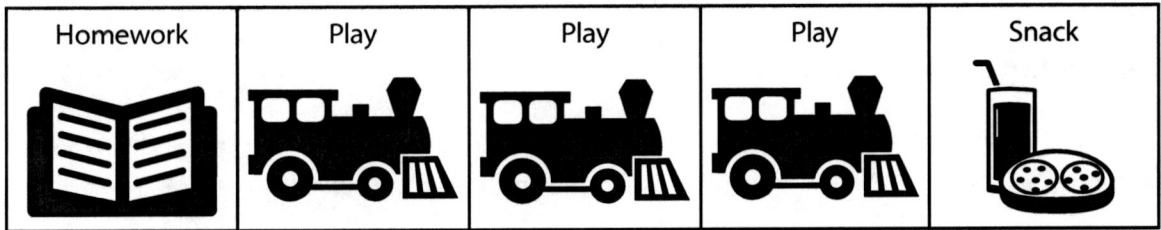

Six-year-old Lucas has a tantrum every time he is asked to do something he doesn't want to do, and especially when it's time to leave a friend's house. The "new rules" for Lucas when he visits his friends are: share, take turns, and leave when mom asks. He is reminded of the rules prior to each visit and is praised for following them during the visit. When it is time to leave, his mother gives Lucas a 10-minute warning and helps him with the clean-up. She reminds him of the rule 5 minutes and again 2 minutes before leaving. When they leave the house, he is praised for following the rules and given a token that can be exchanged for 15 minutes of time to play his favorite game when they get home.

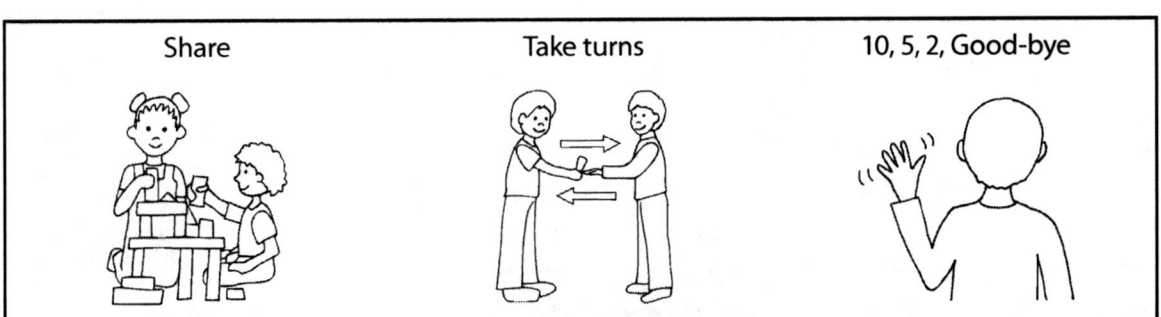

Fixations

Some children with autism develop fixations. A fixation is an obsessive preoccupation. Jack's insistence upon opening and closing the outside doors is an example of a fixation. Usually, the fixation is an interest, activity, or topic that the child enjoys, making it harder to change. Some fixations are manageable, but in other cases, they become extreme and interfere with daily functioning. Adding predictability is usually indicated when fixations become problems.

> *Five-year-old Chang loves to fast forward and rewind his favorite movies. He especially likes to watch Alice go up and down the chute in his favorite movie, "Alice in Wonderland." He can do this for hours and, in fact, does. Every time his parents try to stop him, he screams and cries. The behavior is so frequent and intense that he has broken several DVD players. Whenever his family visits friends, he immediately scopes out their entertainment centers and starts watching movies. Consequences, such as timeout, have met with failure. Chang's parents are at their wits' end trying to figure out what to do.*

✿ Tool: Change the Routine

Again, considering what is reasonable, what fits the Rule of Five, what adds predictability and includes choice, what is the "new" rule? How is it communicated to Chang and what is the new routine?

> *Chang's parents develop new rules regarding watching movies.*
>
> *Chang may ...*
>
> 1. *Watch movies for one hour after school only and one hour on weekends before dinner.*
>
> 2. *He must watch them in the basement family room on a specific player.*

> *They make a visual schedule to communicate the new rules to him. On the schedule is a picture of a school bus, followed by movie in the basement, followed by snack. They explain the new routine in the morning. After school, they show him the schedule again and set a timer for one hour. At the end of the hour, he is shown the schedule and escorted upstairs for snack.*

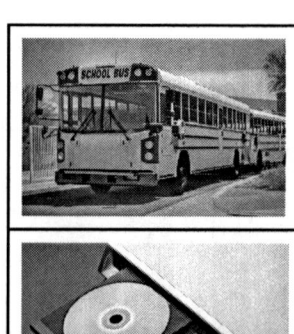

> *Chang is not allowed to watch movies at any other time. His parents are vigilant about the new rules, and after school he is allowed to watch movies immediately. Within one week, Chang has learned the new routine. He doesn't search for movie players when visiting family friends, and he has begun to play with toys and with his sister. The new rules and routine provide him with a predictable time to watch his favorite movies every day. He "knows" that this time is set aside after school, and he trusts that his parents will follow through. After several weeks, without any encouragement from his parents, Chang begins to self-limit movie time to about 10 minutes.*

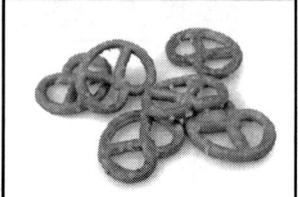

Parent Testimonial:

As a parent with a child on the autism spectrum, each day can be a challenge in so many different ways. My son, Andrzej, is a beautiful 11-year-old former preemie who has gone through a lot medically in his young life. Even though the medical complications have subsided, Andrzej's behavioral issues have persisted. I truly believe his behavioral issues are much harder to deal with than his medical issues.

One issue that we still struggle to manage is Andrzej's propensity for taking his toys apart. Every time he got a new toy, such as a small car, it would be destroyed within a few minutes to a few hours. It was exasperating, So I asked for Judy's help.

We tackled the situation with the following rules and steps:

1. *Andrzej can only play with a new toy when an adult sits right next to him and only for a few minutes.*

2. *Once he proves that he will not take the toy apart, the adult moves behind him but remains in sight of the new toy.*

3. *Next, the adult moves to a different room but stays in sight of Andrzej and the toy.*

4. *Once Andrzej is able to resist the impulse to take a new toy apart, the next step is to purchase a duplicate "practice toy" and allow him to take it to daycare/school.*

If the toy comes home apart, Andrzej has to take an old toy the next day instead. He needs to keep practicing with his old toys until we feel he is ready to try again.

This method was very successful. Andrzej learned that if he wanted to take a new toy to show his friends, he had to make sure he didn't take it apart. We built in rewards along the way. If he received a certain number of stickers, he could buy a duplicate practice toy. Today, Andrzej has a whole bag of new toys that he can play with by himself for as long as he wants. We keep them on a shelf but give him the bag when he asks for it. It is amazing to look back on how many toys we went through. But … it was well worth it!

Lisa Szymanski

Repeated Questions

If your child repeatedly asks the same question(s) about the schedule or fixates on an upcoming event or activity, he may be expressing uncertainty about your answers and feel compelled to check them with you. In other words, he needs reassurance. Giving him a place to check helps with feelings of uncertainty and reduces questioning. Visual supports are often effective in this regard. For example, a calendar showing the schedule of events is very helpful (see Chapter 6); another option is to write out your child's question and your answers in a notebook or on a whiteboard. For questions or topics that persist over days or weeks, a notebook is best. For short-term (day or two) questions, a whiteboard is simpler to use because the questions and answers can be erased and easily replaced as new situations arise. Tell the child to "check the board" or "check your notebook" every time he asks you one of the questions, just like you tell him to "check the schedule." Add new questions and answers as needed. Consistently using this strategy teaches the child where to check for reassurance.

Armed with your box of tools for problem behaviors, let's focus next on how to teach your child new skills. Remember Chapters 4 and 5 when we learned that one of the reasons for a problem is a skills deficit, such as Tom who didn't know how to tie his shoes? This is the focus of the next three chapters – strategies to teach your child the "Now and Forever" rules and social skills, two areas that affect your child's eventual independent functioning.

Action Plan for Chapter 11: Changing Routines and Fixations
(Select From the Choices Below)

Rules to Remember:
- ☐ **If you don't make up the rule, the child may do it for you.**
- ☐ **What is seemingly obvious to others is not obvious to some children with autism.**

Tools to Use:
- ☐ **Come up With a New Rule**
- ☐ **Change the Routine**

To Do:
- ☐ **One new rule is:** _____
- ☐ **The new routine is:** _____

References and Further Reading

Barthold, C. (2013). Environmental engineering/modifications. In F. R. Volkmar (Ed.), *Encyclopedia of autism spectrum disorders* (pp. 1122-1130). New York, NY: Springer Science+Business Media.

Dalrymple, N. J. (1995). Environmental supports to develop flexibility and independence. In K. A. Quill (Ed.), *Teaching children with autism: Strategies to enhance communication and socialization* (pp. 243-264). New York, NY: Delmar Publishers, Inc.

Moskowitz, L. J., Carr, E. G., & Durand, V. M. (2011). Behavioral intervention for problem behavior in children with Fragile X Syndrome. *American Journal on Intellectual and Developmental Disabilities, 116*(6), 457-478.

Chapter 12:
"Now and Forever"

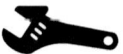

The span of skills needed for independent functioning increases with age and time, and deficits in these areas are often the unrecognized source of challenging behaviors. For example, the skills needed at 5 months are few, while those needed at 5 years of age are numerous, and those at age 25 are countless. As the gap between chronological age and skill development widens, problems can also increase, especially when a child isn't developing new behaviors and skills and negative behavior patterns become entrenched.

We have talked extensively about the Rule of Five throughout this book. It is a critical rule in your Parenting Toolkit and should be a part of most decisions you make regarding your child's future well-being.

Lifelong Skills

The Rule of Five plays a role in accomplishing "now and forever" skills and routines – the independent life skills that don't need to change much with time. Once a child with autism learns to brush his teeth correctly, he can brush his teeth the same way "now and forever." Once he learns to take a shower, load a dishwasher, or sort laundry, he can do it "now and forever" the same way.

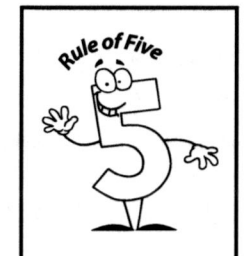

However, unrecognized deficits in these skill areas are often a source of behavior challenges. Parents and other adults sometimes assume a child's misbehavior is willful noncompliance, when in reality it is because the child has not mastered all of the steps to complete a task independently. Some parents assume their child will just naturally, over time, learn the skills needed for independent functioning. Others question how much a child can be expected to learn, and some assume a child can't really learn much at all.

Every child with autism needs help learning the "now and forever" rules and routines. Teaching them is everyone's job, but especially yours as the parent. Don't leave teaching these routines up to your child's school or, worse, believe they will "just happen." Just like every other skill, they must be taught. Some children learn quickly, others need weeks, and maybe months, of repeated practice. Children with autism CAN learn; we just have to teach them.

What's Included?

The skills for lifetime routines are self-help skills like dressing, grooming, and hygiene, and independent skills like eating and food preparation, cleaning, laundry, and shopping. Other lifetime rules and routines include safety rules, such as how to safely cross a street, put on a bicycle helmet, wear a seatbelt in a vehicle, or use a flashlight. Some community skills and routines are "now and forever." For example, how to find a restroom, order from a menu, serve yourself at a buffet, and wait in line. Many social skills, such as greetings, farewells, and checking yourself in for an appointment, can also become lifetime skills.

Getting Started

Although school is a big chunk of every child's day, try to focus on specific lifetime routines for a portion of the remaining hours at home. Concentrate on routines at home and in the community, because you can directly teach and have some control over them.

At this point you may be thinking I'm being unreasonable. Maybe you are exhausted, trying to survive day to day and aren't able to add one more thing to your day. Perhaps you have tried to teach some of the lifetime routines and have run into roadblocks, such as your child's resistance to brushing teeth, to take a bath, refusal to clean up toys, or tantrums when you go out. Perhaps your child is glued to the television, computer, or gaming system and you have given up trying.

Remember, just because you have decided to teach doesn't mean your child is ready to learn. This is why it is important to use all of the rules and tools you learned about in the previous chapters, as well as the new ones below. Let's start with some basic rules.

⚙ Rule: Start teaching early.

Teaching independence must start early. With practice, children as young as 2 years old can throw trash away and carry a bowl into the kitchen after they are finished eating. With guidance and practice, they can learn to put toys and clothes away, hang a jacket on a hook, and use a soap dispenser. Even if your child is engaged in an intensive intervention program for multiple hours a day with therapists in your home, she still has to get dressed, eat, brush teeth, use the toilet, and take a bath. Don't let this precious time to teach routines go to waste. Work on mastering skills and completing them independently.

Many parents tell me that their young children like to "help." My response is, "Wonderful!" Helping is a great social skill, and with lots of practice "helping with a certain task" the child can eventually take over the task and do it independently. Helping routines that involve meaningful activities, such as carrying in and putting away groceries, setting the table, folding laundry (start with wash cloths and hand towels), feeding pets, and clearing the table are great ways to start to learn independence.

> ***My son is 10 years old and still doesn't do many tasks independently. Is it too late?***
>
> Not at all, it is never too late to start teaching! Even if your child is a teenager, begin at whatever age he is right now. The important thing is to get started. You may find it a bit rough at first, because you are changing his current routines and adding new expectations. You also have to find out exactly what he can and can't do. He may have mastered some steps of a task but not all. With an older child, you may have to enlist the support of school staff to help in these assessments and be creative with your reward system. For some older children, an allowance helps.

☼ Rule: Teach the right way from the start.

It takes a child with autism longer to learn skills than typical children. Therefore, to save time and reduce frustration, teach skills the right way from the beginning, including ALL of the steps. One example of where this is important is using the bathroom. Teach your child to close the door. When she is little, toileting with the door open at home is not a big deal; however, when she is 15 and leaves the door open in a public restroom, it is not only awkward but also potentially dangerous.

When you teach the right way from the beginning, you don't have to reteach later. Whatever routines you set up, make sure they fit the Rule of Five. Will they be appropriate in five years? Remember, children with autism are routine-oriented, so the routine will remain for a long time.

☼ Rule: Begin with small and specific tasks.

The number of tasks and skills that your child needs to learn can seem overwhelming at first. For this reason, start with just one or two specific tasks that fit each day's routine circumstances. Typically, a day includes opportunities to focus on skills for dressing, grooming, meals, helping, and social interaction routines. Many youth with autism have difficulty staying organized and managing their time effectively. When you break each day up into chunks and assign various tasks for each time period, you also help them learn to manage their time. Sometimes it is helpful to think about skills and routines for morning, after school, and bedtime.

Illustration 12:1 shows a list of tasks found in three different routines. For example, a morning routine includes tasks such as getting dressed and brushing teeth.

Illustration 12:1 Routines		
Morning Routine	**Staying Safe: Parking Lot Routine**	**Toileting Routine for Girls**
1. Get up. 2. Go to the bathroom. 3. Wash your hands and face. 4. Brush your teeth. 5. Comb your hair. 6. Get dressed. 7. Eat breakfast. 8. Take your medication. 9. Pack your lunch. 10. Put your backpack by the door. 11. Put your shoes on. 12. Get your coat on.	1. Get out of the car. 2. Stand next to the car and wait for the adult. 3. Look for moving cars. 4. Walk next to the adult in the parking lot. 5. Leave store with the adult. 6. Look for moving cars. 7. Walk next to the adult in the parking lot. 8. Wait next to the car. 9. Get into the car. 10. Fasten seatbelt.	1. Enter the bathroom. 2. Close the door. 3. Pull down your pants. 4. Sit on the toilet. 5. Urinate or defecate in the toilet. 6. Take toilet paper and wipe. 7. Pull up your pants. 8. Flush. 9. Wash your hands. 10. Dry your hands. 11. Open the door.

Your child must be able to complete the individual tasks before she can complete the whole routine. Teach the tasks first (and check to make sure she has mastered them), and then focus on teaching the entire routine.

To choose a task, ask your self:

1. Is the task realistic/reasonable given my child's age and current capabilities, or will it be too difficult?

2. Is the task achievable? Can your child learn to perform it successfully with practice?

3. Is the task specific? Will *everyone* who looks at the steps of the task be able to complete it in the same way?

✿ Tool: Self-Help and Independent Skills Checklist

The Self-Help and Independent Skills Checklist in Illustration 12:2 is a comprehensive list of potential "now and forever" skills your child needs for independent functioning. The specific skills or tasks you choose to teach depend upon the age and functioning level of your child. Most tasks have an obvious progression into a routine. For example, taking off and putting on underwear, pants, shirt, socks, and shoes (all individual dressing skills) progress into a dressing routine that eventually includes choosing appropriate clothing that is suitable for the season and weather.

✓ To Do: Complete the Self-Help and Independent Skills Checklist.

Illustration 12:2
Self-Help and Independent Skills Checklist

Check the box that describes your child's current ability to perform the following self-help and independent skills.

Dressing	Cannot do. Requires extensive help.	Can do part. Needs some help.	Can do alone. Does not need any help. May need reminders.	Can do without reminders or help. Completely independent.
Takes off pants (does not include unfastening)				
Puts on pants (does not include fastening)				
Takes off socks				
Puts on socks				
Takes off a pullover shirt				
Puts on a pullover shirt				
Takes off a front-opening shirt or jacket				
Puts on a front-opening shirt or jacket				
Takes off shoes				
Puts on shoes				
Ties shoes				
Zips up a zipper				
Fastens and unfastens buttons and snaps				
Threads a belt				
Buckles a belt				
Hangs up clothes				
Puts clean clothes in a drawer				
Puts dirty clothes in a hamper or basket				
Chooses clothes that match				
Chooses clothes that fit				
Chooses clothes for weather				
Chooses clothes for setting				
Chooses clothes that are clean and in good repair				
Grooming and Hygiene	**Cannot do. Requires extensive help.**	**Can do part. Needs some help.**	**Can do alone. Does not need any help. May need reminders.**	**Can do without reminders or help. Completely independent.**
Uses toilet and toilet paper				
Washes and dries hands				
Washes and dries face				

Washes and rinses body in bath or shower				
Washes and rinses hair				
Dries self after bathing				
Brushes teeth properly				
Combs and brushes hair				
Cleans and trims nails				
Shaves				
Uses a tissue to blow nose				
Uses feminine hygiene products				
Applies deodorant				
Eating, Food Preparation, Clean-Up	**Cannot do. Requires extensive help.**	**Can do part. Needs some help.**	**Can do alone. Does not need any help. May need reminders.**	**Can do without reminders or help. Completely independent.**
Drinks from a cup				
Eats with a spoon				
Eats with a fork				
Spreads with a knife				
Cuts with a knife				
Sets table				
Clears and wipes table				
Pours liquid into cup				
Prepares own snack				
Prepares cold breakfast				
Prepares toast				
Makes a sandwich				
Puts straw into juice box or cup				
Uses a can opener				
Uses measuring cups and spoons				
Follows a written or picture recipe				
Uses microwave				
Uses stove and turns off burners when finished				
Uses oven (sets temperature and timer) and turns off when finished				
Prepares grocery list				
Stores leftover foods				
Discards spoiled foods				
Discards packaging/trash				
Recycles bottles, cans, plastic				
Puts groceries away				

Laundry	Cannot do. Requires extensive help.	Can do part. Needs some help.	Can do alone. Does not need any help. May need reminders.	Can do without reminders or help. Completely independent.
Sorts clean from dirty clothes				
Sorts light from dark clothes				
Strips bed				
Loads and sets washer to correct setting				
Measures soap				
Uses dryer at correct setting				
Hangs up clothes neatly				
Folds clothes neatly				
Puts clothing away				
Cleaning	**Cannot do. Requires extensive help.**	**Can do part. Needs some help.**	**Can do alone. Does not need any help. May need reminders.**	**Can do without reminders or help. Completely independent.**
Puts toys/things away				
Makes bed				
Changes bed linens				
Empties wastebaskets, replaces liner				
Takes out trash				
Dusts furniture				
Sweeps floor				
Vacuums floor				
Washes windows				
Cleans mirrors				
Cleans sink				
Replaces toilet paper roll				
Cleans toilet				
Loads and runs dishwasher				
Unloads dishwasher				
Misc. Home Tasks	**Cannot do. Requires extensive help.**	**Can do part. Needs some help.**	**Can do alone. Does not need any help. May need reminders.**	**Can do without reminders or help. Completely independent.**
Rakes leaves				
Removes snow from sidewalk				
Mows lawn				
Gets mail				
Cares for pets				
Replaces light bulb				

Shopping Skills	Cannot do. Requires extensive help.	Can do part. Needs some help.	Can do alone. Does not need any help. May need reminders.	Can do without reminders or help. Completely independent.
Carries/wears identification				
Shops from written/picture list				
Knows clothing and shoe size				
Recognizes coins and bills				
Uses a debit card				
Keeps money in a wallet				
Follows a map/written directions				
Safety Skills	Cannot do. Requires extensive help.	Can do part. Needs some help.	Can do alone. Does not need any help. May need reminders.	Can do without reminders or help. Completely independent.
Answers the telephone				
Takes phone message				
Safely crosses the street				
Treats a minor cut or burn				
Knows where to go in a storm				
Knows what to do in case of fire				
Knows when and how to call 911				
Knows when and how to lock doors and windows				
Knows when and how to open/close blinds, shades, drapes				
Answers the door and does not let in strangers				
Knows name of doctor and where to locate phone number				
Knows name of dentist and where to locate phone number				
Knows name of nearest urgent care/emergency room				
Knows name and phone number of nearest neighbor				
Takes the right medicine at the right dose at the right time				
Knows own allergies				

Teaching a routine, such as dressing, begins with determining whether or not your child can complete the individual skills that make up the routine with or without help. By completing this skills checklist, you will have a good idea of what your child can and cannot do independently and, therefore, you will know where to start.

1. **Dressing Routines:** If your child doesn't know how to dress himself, start with tasks such as pulling his shirt down or pulling his pants up. If he can dress himself, have him choose appropriate clothes to wear, learn to tie his shoes, zip a jacket, button a shirt, or thread a belt. If he has accomplished all of these dressing-related skills, move towards caring for clothes, such as hanging up clothes, folding and putting them away, or sorting laundry.

2. **Grooming Routines:** Skills in this area include washing hands and face, brushing teeth, combing hair, toileting, and bathing. If your child has accomplished one skill, move on to the next. Children with few sensory issues and good motor control are often able to focus on several skills in this area simultaneously while others may need more support and time.

3. **Meal Routines:** Tasks in this area relate to eating, such as using a fork, cutting or spreading with a knife, and food preparation, such as getting a snack or preparing a cold breakfast. Make meal preparation a family experience by sharing the techniques and responsibilities with everyone in your family; this helps your child learn, too. Assign small tasks, such as measuring or slicing, and work on recipes together as you prepare lunch or dinner. Table manners are very important and will be essential as your child ages. Can your child use a napkin, chew with his mouth closed, and control the pace of eating? Does he respond appropriately when asked to pass a food and have a way to request more of something?

4. **Helping Routines:** Routines in this area are usually related to cleaning up and putting things away after playing, after a meal, or at bedtime. They can also include helping with chores or meal preparation. Helping routines have a beginning and an end, usually follow step-by-step procedure, and once learned correctly, are not forgotten. So be sure and make helping routines a regular part of your child's day.

5. **Leisure and Community Social Routines:** Teaching social interaction skills is the focus of Chapters 13 and 14; however, for purposes of this chapter, be aware that you need to set aside time for social interaction and routines at home and in your community. For example, you may play a game together, take a walk in the park, or go shopping to practice social interaction skills. Perhaps your child is ready to learn and practice telephone skills, such as what to say, how to ask who is calling, and writing down the information for a message.

It doesn't matter what skills and routines you choose to teach, within reason. But remember they must be realistic for your child's age and ability, achievable, and specific. What matters is that you don't leave them to chance. When you select one "job" or task in each of these five areas, you are building your child's abilities one step at a time. As each task is mastered, it becomes a meaningful lifetime skill, part of a routine that doesn't change with age. The more skills your child learns, the more independent he will eventually become.

⚙ Rule: Set the child up to succeed by preparing in advance.

To teach a skill, prepare what you need in advance. Illustration 12:3 details the six antecedents you must think through. These include the materials that are needed (including visual tools), the setting(s) to teach in (put visual tools in each setting that will be used), the context in which to teach, the ideal time(s) to teach, the people who will be responsible for teaching, and the directions for the task.

Illustration 12:3 Tool: Preparing in Advance		
Antecedents	**Description**	**Examples**
1. Materials	Any item needed to teach a skill	Soap, towel, shirt, shoes, visual tool, timer
2. Setting	The place where the skill will be taught	Kitchen, bathroom, bedroom, restaurant, outdoors
3. Context	The relationship between the skill and the need to use it	Breakfast finished = wash hands Get ready for school = get dressed
4. Time	The time needed to teach Establish a "time to begin" phrase	Set aside special practice time or allow extra time when the skill is needed (allow extra time after meals to focus on washing hands) "It's time to …"
5. People	Who will be doing the teaching?	Parents, caregivers, siblings
6. Directions	The steps of the skill, clearly described in visual format (see Chapter 6)	1. Approach sink 2. Turn on water

Parent Testimonial:

We found that our 10-year-old son, Michael, who has autism, responds very well to lists due to his love of the alphabet, words, and reading. If he is upset about a change in his daily schedule or about participating in a new activity, we make a list of steps for the day or activity, and he calms down almost immediately. We also use lists to help him accomplish daily living skills. For example, Michael is learning how to shower independently. A list for that activity might look something like this:

Before Shower

Put in the bathroom: clean washcloth, clean towel, clean underwear, clean clothes

Take clothes off

Put plastic bathmat down in the bathtub

Turn the water to warm

During the Shower

Get in the shower and close the door

Get body, face, and hair wet

Squeeze small drop of shampoo on hand

Rub hands on hair, making bubbles

Rinse hair in water until bubbles are gone

Put bar soap in wet washcloth

Rub washcloth and soap together to make bubbles

Rub soapy washcloth on: face, arms, under arms, neck, stomach, private parts, bottom, legs, feet

Rinse body in water until bubbles are gone

Turn water off

Grab dry towel and get out of the shower

After Shower

Dry off: hair, face, stomach, arms, back, legs

Put on clean clothes

Hang up wet towel

Put dirty clothes in basket

Lists also work well with Michael because he loves to cross off or check off each item as he accomplishes it. His sense of pride when doing so is immeasurable.

Julie, Plymouth, MI

✪ Rule: Use rewards.

The use of rewards was discussed extensively in Chapters 8 and 9. Rewards can make learning a new skill fun; therefore, consider a simple reward that will encourage your young child to keep trying to do what you ask, such as a high five, tickle, or hug. Ideas for rewards are found on the Reward Surveys (see Chapter 8). For older children, learning new skills and tasks is conducive to earning secondary rewards, so don't overlook a token, point, or allowance system. Be sure to praise your child's efforts and set the reinforcement system up in advance.

✪ Rule: Use task analysis and behavior chains.

Most tasks and routines are made up of smaller steps or component parts. Determining these smaller steps is called a task analysis or a behavior chain. Ultimately, these steps become the directions for completing the task, and each step in the chain becomes a cue for the next one. For example, putting toothpaste on a toothbrush becomes the cue to putting the brush in one's mouth. Using a task analysis allows us to teach one step at a time. Some steps involve mini-steps. For example, in order to put water in a cup you have to turn the faucet on and off. Your child may need these mini-steps included in the teaching.

✅ To Do: Complete task analysis.

Think about what you want your child to do, walk through the task, and write down the steps that are involved. Then have someone else complete the activity following your steps to ensure you haven't missed any and to help you determine whether the steps are specific enough. Illustration 12:4 shows the steps in three different tasks – brushing teeth, washing hands, and making a sandwich.

Illustration 12:4 Task Analysis and Behavior Chains		
Brushing Teeth	**Washing Hands**	**Making a Peanut Butter and Jelly Sandwich**
1. Turn on cold water faucet. 2. Put water in a cup. 3. Get your toothbrush. 4. Get the toothpaste. 5. Put the toothpaste on your toothbrush. 6. Brush all of your teeth. 7. Rinse your mouth. 8. Spit. 9. Rinse your toothbrush. 10. Turn off water. 11. Clean up.	1. Approach the sink. 2. Turn on the water. 3. Place hands in the water. 4. Pump soap onto hands. 5. Rub hands together. 6. Rinse hands. 7. Turn off water. 8. Dry hands on a towel.	1. Get the bread. 2. Get the peanut butter. 3. Get the jelly. 4. Get a table knife. 5. Get a plate. 6. Dip the knife in the peanut butter jar and spread it on one slice of bread. 7. Dip the knife in the jelly jar and spread it on the other slice of bread. 8. Put the slices of bread together and place them on a plate. 9. Clean up. Put the bread, jars of peanut butter and jelly away. Wash the knife.

⚙ Rule: Teach one step at a time.

Each step is taught individually in succession, starting with the first step and moving forward (a forward chain), or starting with the last step and moving backwards (a backward chain). My preferred way to teach self-help skills is using a backward chain because the child finishes the task successfully by himself and is quickly rewarded by a sense of accomplishment. We want the teaching session to end in success for the child. When she starts the chain with the first step and you finish it (as with a forward chain, see below), she might feel disappointed and become discouraged because the task doesn't end with her success, but yours. Therefore, my recommendation is that you use a backward chain (see below) when possible.

Prepare the materials and decide how you are going to teach – forward chain or backward chain. Don't forget to make a visual tool of the directions.

✿ Tool: Forward Chain: Brushing Teeth

1. In a forward chain, say the time-to-begin phrase: "It's time to brush your teeth."

2. Point to Step 1, "Turn on cold water."

3. Prompt and guide your child through Step 1 and praise his efforts.

4. Do all of the remaining steps for him.

5. Always start with the same time-to-begin phrase, "It's time to brush your teeth."

6. After the first few practice sessions, let him start Step 1 on his own. Try not to tell him what to do or help him unless it is really necessary (perhaps he doesn't get started, walks away, or does something else).

7. Once he can do Step 1 by himself, point to Step 2, "Put water in a cup."

8. Initially prompt and guide him through Step 2 and praise his efforts.

9. Do all of the remaining steps for him.

10. Once he can do Step 2 without any prompts from you, move on and point to Step 3.

11. As he masters each step in succession, no longer help the child. Do not tell him what to do. You do not want your prompts to become part of the routine. Let him do all of the steps he has mastered on his own. If he really needs help, point to the step. Do only the remaining steps.

✿ Tool: Backward Chain: Brushing Teeth

1. In a backward chain, you teach in reverse order. Say the time to begin phrase: "It's time to brush your teeth."

2. Do Steps 1-8 for your child.

3. Point to Step 9, "Clean up."

4. Prompt and guide your child through Step 9 and praise his efforts.

5. Once he has mastered clean-up, point to Step 8, "Rinse toothbrush."

6. Prompt and guide through Step 8, "Rinse toothbrush," but don't help with Step 9, "Clean up."

7. Praise when he is finished.

8. Always start with the same time-to-begin phrase, "It's time to brush your teeth."

9. Work backwards through all of the steps. As he masters each step in reverse, no longer help him. Let him do all of the steps he has mastered. Do only the remaining steps.

10. To avoid confusion for your child, be sure that everyone who is teaching follows the plans and teaches the steps in the exact same order, whether you are using a backwards or forwards chain.

By the time your child has mastered all of the steps, the only words you say are: "Time to brush your teeth" and your words of praise at the end. And guess what? Your child has mastered a "Now and Forever" skill! Add it to the list of the morning and evening routines. You know it is one skill he can do independently.

✿ Rule: Be consistent and follow through every day.

Once you start to teach a skill, be consistent and follow through every day until the child can complete it by herself. Then require her to do it independently every day as part of her morning, after-school, or evening routine. When skills become part of a daily routine, it is much easier for a child with autism to plan and follow through, because she can anticipate what is expected. It may only take a few days for your child to learn the entire skill, or it may take several weeks. Regardless of how long it takes, when you teach one step at a time, she has an excellent chance of succeeding.

I want to watch my child to make sure she is doing a good job; why can't I stay in the room after she has mastered the skill?

It is fine if you want to stay in the room to encourage her, but be careful. If you insert yourself into the routine, she may expect you to be there all the time. You have spent many hours teaching one step at a time so she can become independent. Why not let her be independent? If you are going to watch, try not to give her directions or prompts of any kind. Remember, teach the right way in the first place. If you don't think your child has completely mastered a step in the skill, it is not yet an independent skill.

How long do we continue to use the visual tool/directions?

Don't get rid of the tool too soon. Keep it in place as long as your child is using it. It is better that your child checks the tool to see what step is next than to ask you, or for you to tell her before she has a chance to ask. That is why you point to the step first, without speaking, and then point again if she needs help. In this way, you teach her to use the tool. Eventually, she won't need it any more and may tell you to put it away. Then you know she is truly independent.

⚙ Rule: Keep track of progress.

The Daily and Weekly Logs in Chapters 2 and 3 can be used to record and monitor your child's progress, or you can develop a different monitoring system. If your child is learning a specific skill, such as hand washing, place a sticky note, arrow, or paper clip on the visual tool next to the step that your child is currently practicing so that everyone knows what step he is working on and which ones he can do by himself (see below). Tape it to your bathroom mirror, laminate it, and tape it to the counter, or place it in a binder near the sink. You can use similar reminder tools in other places of your home for the remaining skills and routines that are being taught.

It is a good idea to mark progress after each teaching session, especially if multiple teachers are involved. Then everyone can consistently follow the plan. A coding system might look like: VP = verbal prompt, PH = physical prompt, PP = picture prompt, IN = independent, AA = adult does it all. For example, the first three steps of brushing teeth might show:

1. Turn on cold water. IN

2. Put water in a cup. PP 🖇 : Currently learning

3. Get your toothbrush. AA

⚙ Rule: Determine reasons for any problems.

Be sure to record any problems. If they persist, you will need to discover the reason for the problem and decide what to do. Perhaps you need to break the skill steps into even smaller steps, choose a different time, or make a change in the environment. Perhaps you need a more powerful reward or a clearer visual tool. Illustration 12:5 lists the variables to consider when reviewing your plan.

Illustration 12:5
Steps to Teaching New Skills

1. Determine the skill to teach.
2. Complete a task analysis (write out the steps of the task).
3. Decide whether to use a backward or forward chain.
4. Develop your reward system (see Chapters 8 and 9).
5. Choose a progress record to monitor success and problems.
6. Develop your visual tool(s).
7. Begin to teach step by step.
8. Fade prompts.
9. If unsuccessful, go back and review Steps 1-8.

⚙ Rule: Create "Now and Forever" routines.

The stressful times at home for children with autism can seem all-encompassing. They include getting ready for school, getting ready for bed, homework, meals, chores, clean-up, interruption of a favorite activity, visitors, schedule changes, and social play. These events can become tense because of the occurrence of an unexpected event (a favorite shirt is in the laundry, more pages of homework than anticipated, or no food the child expects at dinner time), or they are "non-preferred" activities, meaning the child doesn't like to do them, and they may be difficult, requiring academic or social knowledge and skills the child doesn't have. In some cases, these situations are difficult because of rigid routines, such as those discussed in Chapters 10 and 11.

Creating well-planned and predictable daily routines helps to reduce stress. The routines reduce uncertainty and provide more structure to a child's day. They also help your child to develop organizational skills and to manage time, often problem areas for children with autism. Using the visual supports discussed in Chapter 6, develop a master schedule for your child's routines. Illustration 12:6 shows the master schedule for 10-year-old Caleb's school day.

Time	Morning Getting Ready Routine
	Illustration 12:6 **Caleb's School Day Master Schedule**
Time	**Morning Getting Ready Routine**
7:00 a.m.	Get up, go to the bathroom, wash hands and face, get dressed, make bed
7:30 a.m.	Take pills, eat breakfast, brush teeth, backpack by door, shoes on, coat on
8:00 a.m.	School bus
	After-School Routine
4:00 p.m.	Feed Betsy, fix and eat snack (Friday: community helper)
	Empty backpack and organize homework
	Play outside or in the basement when raining (Tuesday: soccer practice)
5:15 p.m.	Dinner helper – assistant chef
	Waiting plan choices: start homework or clean-up, quick game, make lunch, draw
	Eat dinner
	Kitchen clean up
6:15 -	Homework (Friday: family time)
7:15 p.m.	Put homework in backpack
7:15 p.m.	Choice time: TV, computer, iPad, Wii, insect talk, draw, movie, work on photos
	Bedtime, Getting-Ready-for-Tomorrow Routine
8:00 p.m.	Snack, make lunch, pack backpack
	Dirty clothes in laundry, shower, comb hair, put on pajamas, brush teeth
	Set clothes out for tomorrow, read/music
9:00 p.m.	Lights Out

✅ To Do: Develop master schedule for routines.

1. List exactly what you want your child to do on school days and non-school days. If possible, have the child help you make up the list. Essentially, this is an individualized "to-do" list or schedule that includes dressing, grooming, homework, helping activities, meals, and snacks.

2. Divide the tasks into morning, after-school, and evening/bedtime routines (see Illustration 12:6). Include time ranges if your child likes to know the time and can tell time, such as 6:30-7:00: get up, wash face, and get dressed. For children who cannot read or tell time, use pictures or photos to illustrate the tasks and their order.

Get up	Go potty	Wash face & hands	Get dressed	Make bed

3. For some children, it helps to keep the routine in the same order every day; others prefer to choose the order each day. As long as the child has the list to operate from, she shouldn't forget anything. Remember, when activities are predictable, they are less likely to induce stress.

4. The "left-over" time becomes the time for appointments, leisure, and planned social activities or far bigger jobs, such as house cleaning, yard work, or grocery shopping. Label these activities on the master schedule "Home/Community Helper" to help the child understand that this is not "free" time.

5. Social and leisure activities are often the hardest to plan. Try to schedule in time for interactive social activities with others. In the event there are no scheduled activities, this time becomes an unexpected (and most likely pleasing) surprise for the child who can choose what to do with the extra free time (as long as it isn't one of his obsessions/fixations).

6. Schedule time for fixations and restricted interests. If you allow unlimited time or unrestricted access for fixations and obsessions, the child will have serious difficulty stopping the activity to do something else. She will perceive it as an interruption and "taking away" of something she likes and, therefore, might lose control and have a meltdown.

7. One key to success is to plan a child's free time around the expected routines because then it doesn't feel so much like "giving up" something in order to complete another task.

8. One "now and forever" routine to include is "planning for tomorrow," such as organize homework, pack backpack, make lunch, and set out clothes.

9. If your child is not involved in any regular sports activities, add time for exercise or physical activity.

10. School vacations, seasons of the year, and changes in regularly scheduled activities will dictate modifications to the master schedule; therefore, review it regularly with your child and adjust it to accurately reflect what is expected.

11. In addition to the master schedule, use a weekly or monthly calendar for appointments, practices, expected visitors, or any other anticipated events that are not on the master schedule. See Chapter 6 and Illustration 12:7. If you use a computer application, print out an updated calendar every week.

Illustration 12:7 Sample Weekly Schedule						
Sunday	**Monday**	**Tuesday**	**Wednesday**	**Thursday**	**Friday**	**Saturday**
1 10:00 Soccer 1:00 Sam's Birthday party	2	3 4:00 Soccer	4 6:00 School play	5	6 4:00 Community Helper Family Night: Jesse	7 Morning Home Helper 1:30 Hair cut 2:00 Shoe shopping 6:00 Grandma

12. Place both schedules side by side and keep them in a prominent place, such as on a white or corkboard in the kitchen or on the refrigerator. When there is a change in the master schedule, place a sticky note over the spot with the new information. If your child can write, have her write the note and place it where it belongs. Individual copies of the morning and bedtime routines can be kept in a child's room for quick reference. Remember, these routines do not change, they are "Now and Forever."

Note: In Illustration 12:7 "Community Helper" on Friday designates the time for errands and grocery shopping. "Family night: Jesse" confirms that it is Jesse's turn to choose the movie that evening. On Saturday, "Morning Home Helper" shows that chores or other household tasks will be completed during the morning.

I don't think I can do this. I don't like to keep to a schedule, and I don't want my child to become regimented.

I think we agree that you want your child to become independent. That will not happen unless you teach him the skills and give him the tools to be independent. You don't have to keep the schedule the same; you just have to let him know what it is and what your expectations are. By using universal phrases such as Community Helper, Home Helper, or Assistant Chef on the master schedule, you give him advance notice that he will be helping with something. Even if you don't know what you are fixing for dinner until you walk in the door after work, he knows, and you know, that he will be helping with whatever dinner tasks you assign him. Don't make the mistake of giving him nothing to do. Even if you order in pizza, your child can get out the napkins and get glasses for drinks. You do, however, need to keep the Getting Ready routines the same until he has mastered them. Remember, these are "now and forever" routines that set your child up for a lifetime.

In addition to independent skills and "Now and Forever" routines, there is another critical area where your child needs your help. This is the important area of social skills, another area where deficits are often a reason for challenging behavior for children on the autism spectrum. We will turn to those next.

📋 **Action Plan for Chapter 12: "Now and Forever"**
(Select From the Choices Below)

⚙️ **Rules to Remember:**
- ☐ Start teaching early.
- ☐ Teach the right way from the start.
- ☐ Begin with small and specific tasks.
- ☐ Set the child up to succeed by preparing in advance.
- ☐ Use rewards.
- ☐ Use task analysis and behavior chains.
- ☐ Teach one step at a time.
- ☐ Be consistent and follow through every day.
- ☐ Keep track of progress.
- ☐ Determine reasons for any problems.
- ☐ Create "Now and Forever" routines.

✳️ **Tools to Use:**
- ☐ Self-Help and Independent Skills Checklist
- ☐ Preparing in Advance
- ☐ Task Analysis
- ☐ Forward Chain
- ☐ Backward Chain
- ☐ Daily Log
- ☐ Weekly Log

✅ **To Do:**
- ☐ Self-Help and Independent Skills Checklist
- ☐ The "Now and Forever" routine/task is: _____
- ☐ Complete task analysis/behavior chain (Illustration 12:4)
- ☐ Decide forward or backward chain
- ☐ Complete preparations (Illustration 12:3)
- ☐ Choose rewards
- ☐ Develop a master schedule for routines (Illustration 12:6)

References and Further Reading

Adams, J. I. (1997). *Autism-P.D.D. More creative ideas from age eight to early adulthood.* Kent Bridge, ONT, Canada: Adams Publications.

Baker, B. L., & Brightman, A. J. (1989). *Steps to independence: A skills training guide for parents and teachers of children with special needs,* (2nd ed.). Baltimore, MD: Paul H. Brookes.

Cardon, T. A. (2007). *Initiations and interactions: Early intervention techniques for parents of children with autism spectrum disorders.* Shawnee Mission, KS: AAPC Publishing.

Center for Excellence in Developmental Disabilities. *ADEPT autism distance education parent training. Module 1: Strategies for teaching functional skills.* UC Davis Mind Institute. Retrieved from http://media.mindinstitute.org/education/ADEPT/Module1Menu.html

Center on the Social and Emotional Foundations for Early Learning. *Teaching your child to become independent with daily routines.* Vanderbilt University. Retrieved from: http://csefel.vanderbilt.edu/documents/teaching_routines.pdf

Coucouvanis, J. (2008). *The potty journey: Guide to toilet training children with special needs, including autism and related challenges.* Shawnee Mission, KS: AAPC Publishing.

Drahota, A., Wood J. J., Sze, K. M., & Van Dyke, M. (2011). Effects of cognitive behavioral therapy on daily living skills in children with high-functioning autism and concurrent anxiety disorders. *Journal of Autism and Developmental Disorders, 41,* 257-265.

Horner, R. H., Sugai, G., Todd, A. W., & Lewis-Palmer, T. (2000). Elements of behavior support plans: A technical brief. *Exceptionality, 8*(3), 205-215.

Mahler, K. J. (2009). *Hygiene and related behaviors for children and adolescents with autism spectrum and related disorders: A fun curriculum with a focus on social understanding.* Shawnee Mission, KS: AAPC Publishing.

McClannahan, L. E., & Krantz, P. J. (1999). *Topics in autism: Activity schedules for children with autism; Teaching independent behavior.* Bethesda, MD: Woodbine House.

Teaching Social Skills: Part I – Introduction

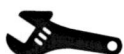

Social skill deficits are another primary reason for challenging behavior. Unfortunately, this often goes unrecognized and remains misunderstood in children with autism. Social skills are not just play skills but include all of the written and unwritten rules of social interaction and behavior. They are complex and often overwhelming.

The goal of teaching social skills is to make positive and lasting changes in your child's personal interaction skills. Ultimately, we want the child to succeed in making friends, sustaining employment, and maintaining an emotionally healthy outlook on life. For this to happen, everyone must assume some responsibility for the teaching and for providing opportunities to practice skills.

⚙ Rule: Social skills require direct teaching, just like other skills.

Social skill deficits don't remit with development or the passing of time. They require directed teaching, just like any other skill. For most individuals with autism, acquisition of social skills is a lifelong challenge. For some, it may be easier. However, every child with autism must transfer skill learning to multiple environments and generalize those skills to each home, school, and community setting. This does not happen automatically. Repetition and persistence are essential. This is the purpose of including Chapters 13 and 14 on selected social skill development in this book, including the following:

- Ask for help
- Ask a question on the topic
- Be a good sport
- Give and receive compliments
- Greet (beginner and intermediate)
- Join in
- Offer encouragement
- Share
- Wait
- Work in a group

⚙ Rule: Teaching is everyone's job, including yours.

Teaching social skills is not just the teacher's job, the speech-language therapist's job, the social worker's job, or the counselor's job. Your child must practice real skills in real-life situations, so every single member of your family must get involved, too. Time is too precious and the skills are too numerous for any one person to teach alone. In fact, social skills are as important as any academic or independent skill you want your child to learn – in fact, they may be more important to your child's eventual outcome. As you learn more about the basics of social skills teaching in this chapter, you will apply this information to the practice tools in Chapter 14.

Discovery

Many years ago I was asked to complete the following activity at a workshop. Take a moment and try it yourself.

1. On a piece of paper, list 10 things you did this morning.

2. Put an "S" next to the items on your list that required social skills.

3. Put an "I" next to the items on your list that required independent skills.

4. Put an "A" next to the items on your list that required academic skills.

The results may come as a surprise to you. Did you have any academic skills on your list? Probably not. This exercise helps confirm the importance of independent and social skills in our every day lives and verifies how small a role that academic skills may actually play.

Sample List
1. Took a shower
2. Got dressed
3. Made breakfast
4. Ate breakfast
5. Packed lunches
6. Checked mail
7. Made a phone call
8. . . .
9. . . .
10. . . .

Social Skill Basics: Fundamental Skills

Eight skills are universal to every social interaction. These are called fundamental skills, and they are shown in Illustration 13:1. Some children with autism have trouble with all of the fundamental skills; others have difficulty with only a few of them.

Illustration 13:1
Fundamental Social Skills

1. *The context:* the who, what, where, when of the situation

2. *Personal space:* how close or far away to be from others

3. *Facial expression:* matching one's facial expression to the circumstances

4. *Voice volume and tone:* how loud or soft to talk for the circumstances; matching appropriate voice tone to the circumstances

5. *Timing:* knowing when to interact or use a specific social skill

6. *Eye contact:* looking at other people

7. *Language:* the appropriate words to say

8. *Actions:* the gestures to use – necessary and appropriate behavior for the situation

---

⚙ Rule: The context determines what skills are needed.

The context of a social interaction typically directs the skills that are needed and how they are used. Being at the library with friends is very different from being at a sporting event. Playing a game with two or three people is different from being on a team. Different skills are required of every setting and circumstance. This is where children with autism often have difficulty.

First, they have to recognize the context and then understand what skills to use. For most of us this is automatic. It's like learning a new language; once we know how to say hello in the new language, we apply that knowledge across all of the situations where a greeting is appropriate in that language. We quickly learn that in some situations greetings are formal, while in others they are informal. However, children with autism might learn the words to use to greet but then not recognize when to use them or how to use them correctly.

> *Oliver is 7 years old. He has a very good memory and can memorize scripts easily, but he is not able to apply them correctly to typical life situations. For example, he shakes hands and says phrases like "have a good weekend" even when it is not Friday.*

⚙ Rule: Fundamental skills are integrated parts of other skills.

For example, a group of children are playing a game of tag at the park. This is the *context*. Some of the skills necessary for this social interaction include greeting, joining in, being a good sport, and offering encouragement. Handling teasing, waiting, and dealing with disappointment might also be required. *Personal space* will likely change when each of these skills is used. Each child's *voice tone and volume* may change as the game progresses and becomes more exciting. At the same time, each child will need to remember to use appropriate tone and volume when tagged *(timing)*. Facial expressions *(including eye contact)* will change throughout the game as each child is tagged or not. If a child is tagged frequently (or never chased), he will need to be a good sport – by *acting* appropriately and using appropriate *language*.

The interrelationships of the skills, coupled with the constantly changing "rules," make learning social skills very tough. When you consider the thousands of potential social situations, and the fact that your child will not automatically apply what he learns in one setting to another, you can begin to understand how critical it is that all of us get involved.

❀ Tool: Super Skills

The *Super Skills* (Coucouvanis, 2005) approach identifies specific social deficits unique to each child and teaches appropriate prosocial behavior one step at a time. Each social skill is subdivided into separate actions or characteristics that are easy for a child to practice methodically. These steps are called the Steps to Success. For example, the basic steps to "ask for help" are:

1. Recognize you need help.
2. Think of who can help.
3. Move close to the person.
4. Say the person's name.
5. Ask in a friendly voice.
6. Say: "Thank you."

With time, children recognize that some actions are present in most social interactions ("use a friendly voice" or "look at the person"). Although skills are taught one at a time, it quickly becomes apparent that they are interrelated. There are three types of skills in the *Super Skills* program:

1. Social initiation skills
2. Social response skills
3. Getting along with others.

Examples of each are shown in Illustration 13:2. *Social initiation skills* involve approaching another person to start a communication or social interaction. *Social response skills* are used in response to a communication or interaction initiated by someone else, or in response to an event in the environment. *Getting along with others* includes the reciprocal skills necessary to generate positive relationships. They require being able to adjust personal behavior to relate to what another person is saying or doing.

	Illustration 13:2 *Super Skills*	
Social Initiation	**Social Response**	**Getting Along With Others**
Greeting	Replying to greetings	Cooperating
Meeting new people	Answering questions	Compromising
Giving a compliment	Following directions	Negotiating
Asking for help	Using manners	Being a good sport
Joining in a conversation	Staying on task	Showing interest in others
Using proper names	Waiting	Being flexible
Inviting a peer to play/join in	Giving encouragement	Dealing with teasing
Starting a conversation	Reading body language	Receiving a suggestion

Super Skills was originally designed for use in a group but have been modified for your use here. The activities can be used by anyone, including parents, support staff, neighbors, extended family, siblings, and peers, all of whom can facilitate successful achievement of appropriate social behavior, and all of whom can be recruited to help transfer learning into real-life circumstances.

There is no one universal approach to teaching social skills. In fact, there are a variety of approaches for you to explore. Other tools, such as video modeling, story formats, group teaching, peer modeling, and others that you may read about, are not included in this chapter. However, sources for learning about them are listed in the resource section at the end of the book.

✿ Rule: Social skill deficits are one reason for challenging behavior.

Most of the skills included in this chapter are basic skills; they are the foundation for more complex skills. Deficits in these basic skills are often one of the unrecognized reasons for challenging behaviors.

Suppose a child confidently greets her teacher every day but doesn't greet classmates, grandparents, or friends, even when they greet her; in fact, sometimes she says, "Go away" upon meeting somebody. This child has not mastered the social skill of greeting. She may know the component parts, such as eye contact and tone of voice, but she has not mastered the related rules of greeting; that is, when someone greets you, it's polite to greet them in return and it is impolite to tell friends and grandparents to "go away." She is not recognizing the need to use the skill in context.

What Is Mastery?

In this book, mastery means a person knows when and how to use a skill appropriately and with confidence in multiple environments. The skill has become a valuable "habit."

✪ Rule: Identify specific skills for focused teaching.

Identifying specific skills to teach is an essential component of *Super Skills,* and one that I encourage you to use. When you identify a specific skill or set of skills for your child to work on, then everyone is focused on the priority social skills for your child. Without such a focus, the teaching becomes haphazard, and your child's social deficits can seem hopelessly overwhelming. Mastery of the specific skills you have identified temporarily takes precedence over other social deficits, which become of secondary importance. In this way, one step at a time, progress occurs and your teaching efforts don't seem futile. Once skills are achieved, or sufficient progress has been made so that everyone agrees they are no longer a priority, new skills are selected.

✿ Tool: Social Skill Daily Practice Log

The Social Skill Daily Practice Log (Illustration 13:3) is a tool to help you select the skill(s) to work on and keep track of how your child is working on the skill and her progress. Your child can also use the tool to independently monitor her own progress. The Social Skills Daily Practice Log lists all of the skills included in Chapter 14. Certainly, you can modify the tool to include other skills as these are mastered. If you are not sure how your child interacts in other social environments, ask your friends, relatives, and the child's teachers.

Choose one to three skills to work on. You want your child to be successful, so start with skills that show potential to grow and develop. Consider starting with skills that your child …

1. Uses in some social environments, but not all
2. Uses with some people, but not everyone
3. Uses partially consistently (uses some steps but not all)
4. Is frustrated by and that, therefore, are the reason for challenging behaviors in social environments
5. Identifies as important

Illustration 13:3
Social Skills Daily Practice Log

Week of _____

Mark the skills to be practiced for the week. Write the skill number that was practiced under the Day of the Week. Describe the activities that were performed. Add any comments or ideas for new activities to try. Finally, in the last column, record progress with one, two, or three plus signs (see page 171).

1. Ask Questions on the Topic	2. Ask for Help	3. Be a Good Sport	4. Give, Receive Compliments	5. Greet	6. Join In	7. Offer Encouragement	8. Share	9. Wait	10. Work in a Group
Day of the Week				**Skill Activities**			**Comments, Questions, Other Ideas**		**Progress**
Sunday									
Monday									
Tuesday									
Wednesday									
Thursday									
Friday									
Saturday									

Carl, age 10, occasionally greets the principal at school. Greetings are relatively straightforward, and he has lots of neighbors and family members to practice with, so greetings are selected as focus for more teaching and practice. Carl likes to talk about his special topics but doesn't know how to join in on the topic that others are talking about so that is chosen as the second skill. Finally, he willingly shares treats with visitors but doesn't recognize that he needs to share his toys too, so that is the third skill.

Shayene, age 4, has very limited language. She knows how to wave and say "bye." She also uses single words for "no," "milk," "juice," and "cheese" and some word approximations to communicate. Some of her speech is echolalic (she repeats what others say). She claps hands and smiles. Her parents decide to focus on greeting. Shayene already knows how to wave, so they begin to require that she raise her hand in greeting and start to say "hi" when she gets up in the morning, after school, and when they visit family members. Because Shayene knows how to clap, they start to encourage her to watch her brother shoot baskets and clap when he succeeds, preparing her to accompany them to his basketball games and cheer his successes.

What can I do if my child has mastered the skills in this book?

If your child has mastered all of the skills in this book, move on and explore the full *Super Skills* curriculum and the other social skill resources at the end of this book for more suggestions for specific skills to teach. References for assessment tools are also included.

❋ Tool: Skill Steps (See also Chapter 14)

For each skill there is a list of suggested steps, called Steps to Success. These explain what behaviors the skill consists of when used appropriately. When you are teaching a skill, post these steps in a prominent place, such as on the refrigerator or in your child's bedroom or play area. Also, keep a copy in the glove compartment of your vehicle or on your smartphone for use when you are out and about. Posting the steps is a visual tool to help your child remember what to do and how to do it. Pictures can accompany the words if needed. Some examples are included in Chapter 14. Remember, visual tools remind everyone of the expectations.

The steps included with each skill can be modified to fit your child more specifically. In some cases, the steps need to be simplified, in other cases more complex language can be added. An example is shown in the skill for greeting. Note the Beginner Steps and the Intermediate Steps.

Review the steps daily with your child. Explain what the words mean if necessary; show your child how to act out each step and then suggest he try. Talk about how he is going to practice that day and set up a goal for the number of trials.

Teaching social skills may provoke anxiety in your child and fear of failure may be compelling. Asking a child with autism to "try" an unfamiliar activity where there is a chance of error frequently increases stress. So be prepared, be positive, try to make the learning fun, and model positive self-talk, such as "I can do this. I'll be OK."

✿ Tool: Use Rewards

Offering incentives to motivate your child to try a skill, perhaps by earning points or tokens that can be exchanged for small prizes, is one way to encourage practice. (See Chapters 8 and 9 for more information about using rewards.) If you decide to use rewards, remember to reduce the frequency of rewards as your child becomes more skillful. For example, initially you might reward the child every time he shares his toys, but after a few days you might reward after an hour or two of "good sharing." After a couple of weeks, reward only after a whole day of appropriate sharing.

The Social Skills Daily Practice Log is another way to monitor your child's efforts to practice skills and to reward his efforts. The final column is used to record progress with one, two, or three plus signs. The purpose is to rate effort, not perfection, so even if your child does poorly, he should receive some credit. If possible, encourage self-monitoring and have your child rate his own progress.

For older, or more skilled children, discuss progress at the end of the week and set goals for the next week. Your child might like to choose a reward to work towards the following week, such as "home movie night," a slumber party, or a visit with a friend or family member.

✿ Tool: Modeling (See also Chapter 14)

Notice that modeling the skill for the child in natural circumstances is a listed activity for every skill. Remember, your child may be a visual learner. That is, she learns by what she "sees," so you and others can help her learn by showing her exactly what to do.

✿ Tool: Practice Activities (See also Chapter 14)

For each skill there are also suggestions for how to practice it. You will likely have your own ideas, too. Write your ideas on the Social Skills Daily Practice Log so that you can share them with others. It is essential that you actively search for multiple opportunities to use the skill and rehearse with your child in advance if necessary. Don't leave the development of social interaction skills to chance. In fact, plan social skill time equal to homework time. Your child must have social experiences if he is going to develop skills. The more situations in which your child practices a designated skill, the greater the likelihood he will add it to his permanent repertoire. Remember that just because he has learned to play a specific game with you at home, he will not automatically know how to play it with friends or at a relative's house. He needs your help.

Your job as a parent includes orchestrating well-structured situations for social interaction, anticipating problems, and being prepared to actively model, facilitate, coach, and encourage your child. Don't invite friends over to play with your child and then ignore them. Set up activities and plan out the time together with your child in advance, talk about the "what ifs" and how you will manage them together. Over time, as your child is successful, very slowly fade yourself into the next room. Too often, parents take a passive role from the start, assuming the child will "figure it out." For children with autism, this isn't helpful, because they don't have the skills to "figure it out" on their own. You have to show them what to do. So get involved and help ensure the social experience be positive for everyone.

Guided practice involves advance planning. Sit down with your child ahead of time and answer the following questions. Pretend you are your child's friend and act out what to do. Make a written plan that your child can review multiple times if necessary.

**Guided Practice
Receiving Friends/Visitors**

1. What do I say when my friend arrives?
2. What will we do?
3. Make a plan (use pictures, photos, diagrams, or drawings if needed).
4. Who decides what to do?
5. What do I do if we need help or there is a disagreement?
6. What do I say when my friend leaves?

🔧 Rule: Emphasize the positive, not the negative.

A dangerous mistake when working with your child in the presence of others is to be overly critical and focus on her shortcomings. While it is true that your child may have to be reminded of her errors, don't dwell on her mistakes. When correction is needed, it is more effective to tell the child what to do. For example, if your child is supposed to greet and she forgets to say "hi," instead of correcting her by saying, "You forgot to say hi," say, "I'm glad you smiled at Grandma; let's say hi, too." Similarly, if your child is supposed to share, instead of saying, "Don't take all the blocks," say, "Please give some blocks to Sander." In this way, your child is encouraged to try once more.

🔧 Rule: Arrange for practice opportunities at home.

In the course of a day, there are many opportunities for social interaction. Take advantage of them! Although all of us need some time to ourselves, don't let your child hibernate in his room. Sometimes we think we are doing a child a favor by setting up a personal entertainment center in his bedroom, complete with television, DVD, computer, and game systems. This is great for babysitting, but none of these electronics will help your child master social interaction. For that to happen, he has to interact with real-live people in real-life settings. As hard as it is, I suggest one television, one main computer, and one DVD player in the household. That way everyone has to negotiate, share, and compromise.

Another natural opportunity to practice skills is during mealtime. I realize that many families don't sit at the table and eat together, unless eating in a restaurant. Everyone has different schedules, food preferences, and eating habits. Even so, try to have at least one other person eat at the same time as your child with autism and try to eat together as a family at least two or three times a week. Plan and prepare those meals together. Additional suggestions for promoting social interaction at home are shown in Illustration 13:4 and in Chapter 14.

Illustration 13:4
Promoting Social Learning at Home

☐ Play board games, card games, and outdoor games by the rules, and don't "let" your child "win." Model being a good sport by saying, "Good game," or "Maybe I will win next time."

☐ Require that siblings work together to complete a chore, project, activity, or task, such as setting or clearing the table, folding laundry, making a bed, carrying in groceries, baking cookies, preparing a pizza, or making a birthday card for a family member.

☐ Practice popular recess games and activities at home. Teach the rules as well as competence.

☐ Promote interaction by supplying a limited number of materials for some activities, such as decorating cupcakes, dying eggs, making pizza, playing with clay, or playing in the sand box, thus creating a need to share, take turns, ask, or trade with others.

☐ Limit electronics, including TV and computer time.

☐ Watch television together without the sound and practice reading facial expressions.

☐ Have parties several times a year and invite your child's friends and classmates so that you can get to know them and they get to know each other. Explain how to handle any unusual behaviors. Perhaps you want the friend to come and get you if your child starts spinning objects or hits his head with his fist and you are not right there. Find out their birthdays and have your child send birthday greetings.

☐ Skype or video call family members and friends, and have your child join in. Practice in advance what he will talk about or show.

⚙ Rule: Arrange for practice opportunities in the community.

Community activities are prime settings to learn the rules for social interaction and offer a gold mine of opportunities to practice. Take your child with you when you go shopping, eat out, or run errands. Take your child to the park, to the library, to a movie. See Chapters 11 and 12 for tools to use if you and your child have problems in public. Initially, you may have to keep the visits short so your child can be successful.

Enrolling your child in Scouts, clubs, team sports, sports lessons, and art and drama activities is often an option in many communities. Some organizations may offer scholarships or your local autism foundation may provide financial assistance. Besides, many activities are free or low cost, such as taking walks, going for a hike, or riding a bike (some communities offer lessons for children with special needs).

Arrange visits with family, friends, and neighbors. Network with them to set up more opportunities for your child in the community. Think about how to set your child up to be successful; if you are going to visit a friend, take along a game that he already knows how to play. If you are going to the park, bring some toys for the sand box, a bat and ball, or a soccer ball. If you are going to the lake, bring beach toys along.

⚙ Rule: Teach "Now and Forever" social rules.

"Now and Forever" social rules are those that typically don't change with time or circumstances. Sometimes these rules are referred to as the "hidden curriculum" (see Chapter 7). Often persons with autism don't automatically recognize and understand them. Examples of these rules include:

- Don't tell someone next to you that she is fat.

- When someone greets you, it is polite to greet in return.

- Say, "excuse me" when you accidentally bump into someone.

- Go to the end of a line, not the front or the middle.

- Say, "no thank you" if you do not want a food that is offered to you.

- Say," thank you" when you receive a gift, whether you like it or not.

Before you reprimand your child for a social mistake, determine if she truly understands the rule. It is quite likely that she doesn't, so you will need to teach her. Learning the "now and forever" social rules can appear overwhelming. There are more resources to help you and your child at the end of the book.

Children with autism have social and other skill deficits. Teaching the appropriate skills and desirable behaviors is one of your primary jobs as a parent. Therefore, focusing your efforts on teaching appropriate behaviors and skills rather than reacting to misbehavior will likely be more helpful to your child in the long term. She needs your help. Chapter 14 will guide your efforts to teach 10 basic skills that are typically problem areas for children with autism.

Action Plan for Chapter 13: Teaching Social Skills Part I
(Select From the Choices Below)

Rules to Remember:
- ☐ Social skills require direct teaching, just like other skills.
- ☐ Teaching is everyone's job, including you.
- ☐ The context determines what skills are needed.
- ☐ Fundamental skills are integrated parts of other skills.
- ☐ Social skill deficits are one reason for challenging behavior.
- ☐ Identify specific skills for focused teaching.
- ☐ Emphasize the positive, not the negative.
- ☐ Arrange for practice activities at home.
- ☐ Arrange for practice activities in the community.
- ☐ Teach "now and forever" social rules.

Tools to Use:
- ☐ Social Skills Daily Practice Log
- ☐ Skill Steps
- ☐ Rewards
- ☐ Modeling
- ☐ Practice Activities

To Do:
- ☐ First skill to teach: _____ Where:_____ Who:_____
- ☐ Second skill to teach: _____ Where:_____ Who:_____
- ☐ Third skill to teach: _____ Where:_____ Who:_____

References and Further Reading

Bixler Coffin, A., & Hudson, J. (2007). *Out and about: Preparing children with autism spectrum disorders to participate in their communities.* Shawnee Mission, KS: AAPC Publishing.

Coucouvanis, J. (2005). *Super skills: A social skills group program for children with Asperger Syndrome, high-functioning autism, and related challenges.* Shawnee Mission, KS: AAPC Publishing.

Koegel, L. K., & LaZebnik, C. (2004). *Overcoming autism: Finding the answers, strategies and hope that can transform a child's life,* New York, NY: Penguin Books.

Loomis, J. W. (2008). *Staying in the game: Providing social opportunities for children and adolescents with autism spectrum disorders and other developmental disabilities.* Shawnee Mission, KS: AAPC Publishing.

Myles, B. S., Trautman, M. L., & Schelvan, R. L. (2013). *The hidden curriculum for understanding unstated rules in social situations for adolescents and young adults* (2nd ed.). Shawnee Mission, KS: AAPC Publishing.

Pratt, C., & Buckmann, S. (2002). Ten steps towards supporting appropriate behavior. *The Reporter, 7*(3), 24-28. Retrieved from http://www.iidc.indiana.edu/index.php?pageId=469

Weiss, M. J., & Harris, S. L. (2001). Teaching social skills to people with autism. *Behavior Modification, 25*(5), 785-802.

Chapter 14:
Teaching Social Skills: Part II – The Tools

This chapter presents the tools to teach 10 basic social skills: Ask for Help, Ask a Question on the Topic, Be a Good Sport, Give and Receive Compliments, Greet (beginner and intermediate), Join In, Offer Encouragement, Share, Wait, and Work in a Group. Specifically, it includes the steps to the skill both in written and in an alternative picture format, an explanation of the skill, and suggested practice activities. Remember that you can modify the steps by making them simpler or more complex to fit your child's specific learning needs. For additional instructions on how to use these materials and more ideas for how to teach social skills, see Chapter 13. (Much of the information presented here is from my book *Super Skills*, 2005.)

Skill 1: Ask for Help

It is OK to ask for help. Sometimes other people have different ideas and information that might help to make the task easier.

To ask for help, you:

1. Recognize you need help.

2. Think of who can help.

3. Move close to the person.

4. Say the person's name.

5. Ask in a friendly voice.

6. Say: "Thank you."

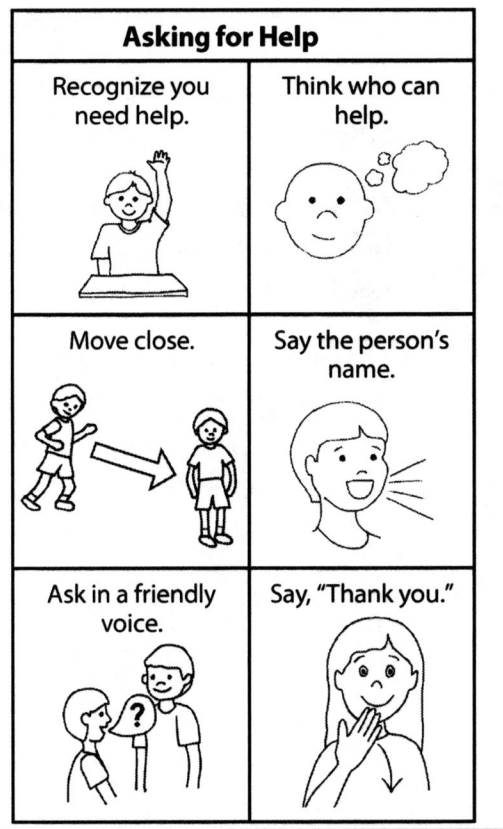

Asking for help is frequently very difficult for children with autism. Some prefer to figure things out for themselves and may view asking for help as personal failure. Others don't consider asking for help an option. They don't recognize that another person might have information or skills different from their own and, therefore, be useful to them. In addition, it is often difficult to accept mistakes – both in themselves and in others – so asking for help becomes even more difficult because what if the other person is "wrong."

Set up situations and activities that require help. The emphasis in teaching this skill is helping your child:

- Recognize when help is needed
- Know that it is permissible to ask for help
- Figure out whom to ask and what to say
- Recognize asking for help does not mean one is a failure

✿ Tool: Practice Activities

1. Set up helping activities every day. Emphasize helping rather than chores (see Chapter 12). Model how to ask for help throughout your daily routines. Ask your child to help you with a task or household project. Make sure you explain to your child why you need help – the task will get done faster, it takes two people, the task is too hard, etc.

2. Look for opportunities for the child to practice offering to help others, such as younger siblings, grandparents, neighbors, etc.

3. Prompt the child to ask for help when you see she needs help with a problem or an activity. Encourage asking for help.

4. Deliberately orchestrate situations where your child will most likely be required to ask for help in order to complete a task you assign. Ideas: turn the mattress on your bed, carry a heavy box, carry in groceries, find a particular movie or library book, bake a cake.

5. Talk about how people help each other daily. Point out instances of people helping each other as you observe them – perhaps someone holding a door open at the store, carrying packages, looking for a lost item, etc.

Skill 2: Ask a Question on the Topic

When you ask a question on the topic, you ask about the same subject that others are discussing.

To ask a question on the topic, you:

1. Listen.

2. Ask yourself: "What are people talking about?"

3. Wait until the other person stops talking.

4. Look at the person.

5. Ask a question about the same thing others are talking about.

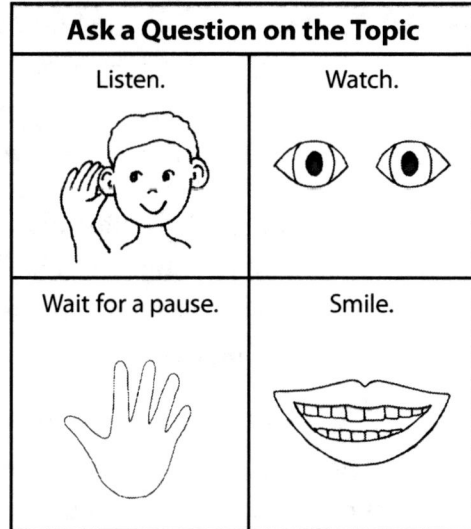

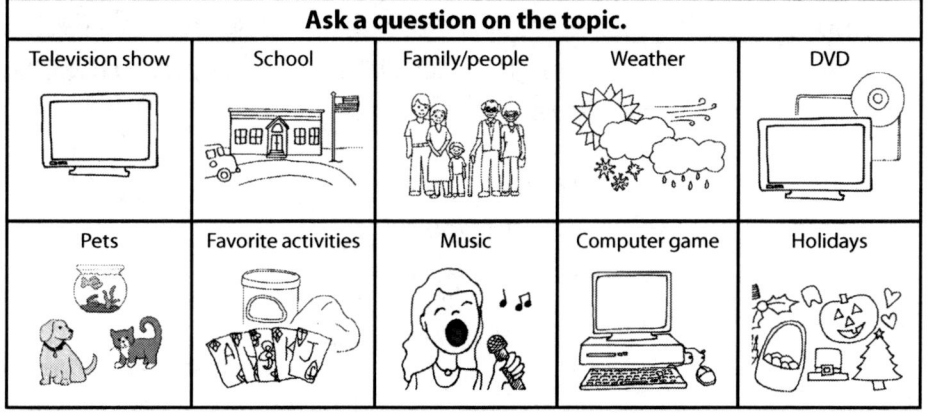

The purpose of this skill is to join a conversation by talking about the same things that others are talking about. This can be difficult, but is very important when interacting with others. The most difficult part for children with autism is to wait for a pause and to join in on the topic.

🌸 Tool: Practice Activities

1. Begin a conversation topic library. Write out questions about any specific topic on 3x5" note cards (one question per card). You may decide to color code the cards (e.g., vacation in red, school in blue). Divide the cards up among those participating (this is a great dinner activity). Start with two or three exchanges on the topic. Practice looking at and reading the 3x5 cards if necessary. (This will seem stilted and unnatural at first, but the child will soon learn what to say without looking.) The idea is to join in at the right time with an appropriate question. Praise the child for joining in. Make the pauses between questions/comments longer than usual so the child has ample time to "join in." Prompt and cue as necessary; by touching your child's card, nodding your head while looking straight at your child or, if necessary because your child does not join in, saying, "your turn." Once the child learns a particular conversation routine, use it at other times of the day in more natural settings.

2. If your child regularly joins in conversations "off the topic," prompt with: "Ask something on the topic," "The topic is _____ now," or "That's not on the topic now, ask something on the topic." Do not answer the child's question or talk to the child on the child's topic and thereby reinforce the behavior. You may need to set up a specific time of the day to talk about the child's special topic of interest. This often helps when the child's topic is a fixation, or obsessive interest.

3. If your child consistently interrupts, label the behavior, such as "That's interrupting. Please wait for a pause" or "wait your turn" and hold up your hand in a "wait" signal. Put your hand down when it is OK for the child to talk. It may be helpful to say, "I'm talking; please wait your turn." And when you are finished talking say, "OK, your turn to talk."

4. If your child monopolizes the conversation, use the "10-second, 10-word rule." Your child must make comments/ask questions in 10 words within 10 seconds or less. Use a timer or count if necessary. Cut the child off when she has exceeded the limit.

5. Prompt your child to join in conversations as the opportunity arises. It may help to carry a stack of possible conversation comments/questions and simply hand the child an appropriate card. Gradually fade the use of the cards.

6. Role play possible conversations ahead of time; offering suggestions of what your child might ask at a party, at grandmother's, at a restaurant, etc.

Skill 3: Be a Good Sport

Sometimes you win and feel happy. Sometimes you lose and feel disappointed. It's OK. Everyone tries to be a good sport when they lose.

To be a good sport, you:

1. Keep a friendly face and voice.

2. Take a deep breath to stay calm.

3. Think: "I'm disappointed, but I can handle this."

4. Make a plan: Congratulate the other players. Say, "Good game." Think, "Maybe next time."

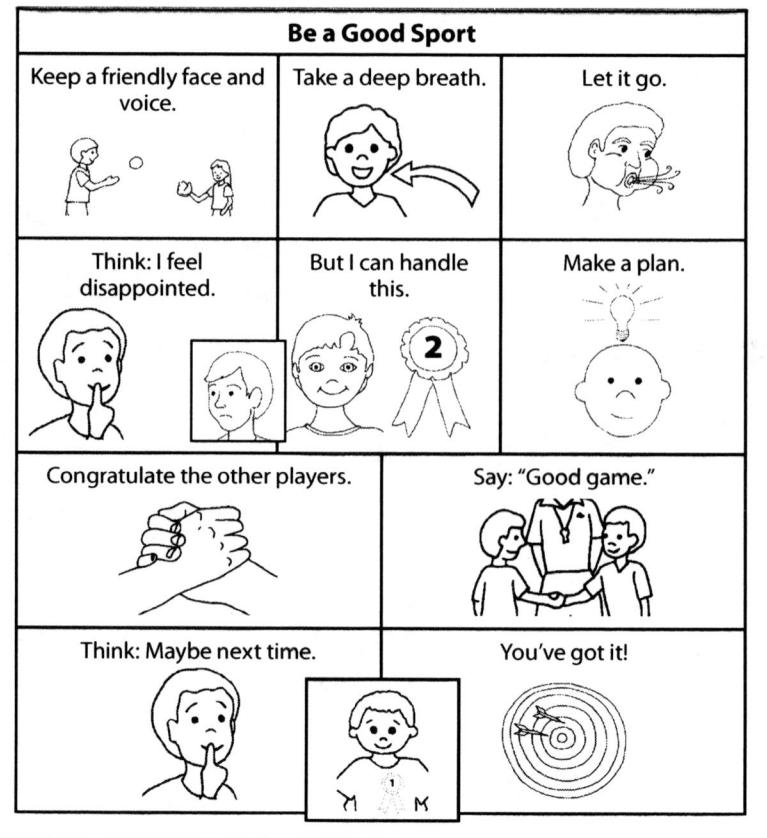

Be a Good Sport

Keep a friendly face and voice.	Take a deep breath.	Let it go.
Think: I feel disappointed.	But I can handle this.	Make a plan.
Congratulate the other players.		Say: "Good game."
Think: Maybe next time.		You've got it!

When a competitive situation is especially difficult or frustrating, it is hard for most children to be good sports. For children with autism, the difficulty often lies in the unpredictable nature of competition. Sometimes you win – sometimes you lose. When a child expects to win, not lose, and he relies on routines to cope, the unpredictability of competition can be especially traumatic. Sometimes losing is perceived as failure and being "wrong." In other cases, the child cannot predict the actions of others, so how can he predict that someone else might win? Some children would rather leave a game than finish it when they see they are losing. Some prefer not to play in the first place because they might lose. Many react to disappointment by crying, screaming, or becoming aggressive.

Structured teaching in good sportsmanship is essential. You cannot simply remove your child from all competitive activities or shelter him by always "letting him win." Although losing may be disappointing, it is not the end of the world. We must work with our children to develop self-control, good sportsmanship, and flexibility so they can develop the skills necessary for positive social interaction.

❀ Practice Activities

1. Play games by the rules. Don't allow your child to cheat in order to win. Always play the correct way. Don't allow your child to leave a game because she is losing. It is OK to take a short break, but insist that the game be completed. Consider rewarding the person who loses.

2. If your child typically handles losing by becoming upset, don't set her up to win to prevent an outburst. Rather, expose her to more situations where she loses. That way she will eventually learn that losing is not the end of the world. Model being a good sport by saying, "Good game" or "Maybe I will win next time." Consider rewarding your child for being a good sport.

3. Use natural situations to be a good sport, such as with difficult tasks and frustrating experiences. Prompt as needed.

4. Praise your child whenever she spontaneously handles disappointment well, such as letting someone else go first, handling losing, saying "good game," etc.

5. Point out whenever you or someone else is being a good sport. Also, point out poor sportsmanship in others and ask your child what the other person might do or say to be a good sport.

6. Consider starting a marble jar to help demonstrate good sportsmanship and/or handling of disappointment. Each time the child is a good sport, she is congratulated and receives a marble for the jar. As the jar fills, she is reminded of how well she is doing.

Skill 4: Give and Receive Compliments

A compliment is a gift to someone. It makes the person feel good. To give a compliment, you:

1. Look.

2. Use a friendly face.

3. Use a sincere voice and say the person's name.

4. Say what you like about what the person did.

To receive a compliment, you:

1. Smile.

2. Look.

3. Say, "thank you."

Giving and Receiving Compliments	
To give a compliment:	
Look.	Use a friendly face.
Use a sincere voice.	Say what you like about what the person did. You are fun.
To receive a compliment:	
Smile and look.	Say: Thank you.

A compliment is something nice one says about another person. When compliments are sincere, they can mean a lot to the people who receive them. Compliments can address aspects of another's personality, skills or talents, or the way a person looks, such as "Jeff, you really worked hard on that math assignment" or "I like your haircut, Amy." When children have difficulty taking another person's point of view, as is often the case for children with autism, they may not see the value of giving compliments in developing friendships. They may not recognize that giving a compliment helps the child to be viewed as a friendly, positive person. Teach that giving compliments is being friendly. Equally important, teach the child to recognize and acknowledge compliments with "thank you" rather than "I know that."

🌸 Practice Activities

1. Write the names of family members on pieces of paper and put them into a container. At mealtime, have everyone choose a name and think of a compliment to give the person they chose. Practice both giving and receiving the compliments.

2. On special holidays that honor family members, such as Grandparent's Day, Mother's Day, Father's Day, and birthdays, have the child think of a compliment to give the honoree and write it out in his best handwriting or on the computer. Have the child decorate the paper and put it into a decorated envelope or box. Put a nametag on the present and exchange the gift.

3. If your child has difficulty thinking of compliments, write out suggested compliments on 3x5 cards ("I like your sweatshirt." "Great cookies." "You are really kind"). Have the child decide to whom to give the compliment and then reward him for doing so.

4. Play board games using compliment cards (see below); in order to spin or throw the dice, one must choose a phrase and say it in a sincere voice with a friendly look.

5. Write compliments, such as those suggested below, on wooden craft sticks and place them in a jar or other container. Label the jar "Smileys." When friends or family members visit, have your child pick a smiley from the container and say it.

I'm glad you are here today.	I like it when you . . .	You are fun to be with.
You have good ideas.	I'm glad you're here.	You make me smile.
You are a good friend.	It's fun knowing you.	I'm glad we're together.
It is good to see you.	You are nice.	I like to work with you.
I like the way you . . .	I like you.	It's fun being together.
I like knowing you.	Thank you for . . .	I like playing with you.
You are friendly.	You are great.	You are really good at . . .

Skill 5: Greet (Beginner Steps)

When you enter a place and see someone you know, when you meet someone new, or when someone greets you, it is polite to say hi.

To greet someone, you:

1. Smile.

2. Look at the person

3. Say, "Hi."

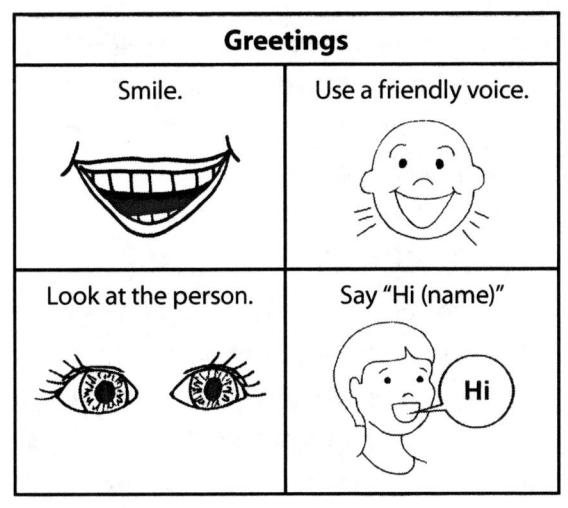

Greetings	
Smile.	Use a friendly voice.
Look at the person.	Say "Hi (name)"

Skill 5: Greet (Intermediate Steps)

When you enter a place and see someone you know, when you meet someone new, or when someone greets you, it is polite to say hi.

To greet someone, you:

1. Use a friendly face and voice.

2. Look at the person.

3. Keep a calm body.

4. Greet the person by saying something like "Hi," "Hello," or "How are you?"

5. Say their name if you know it.

Greeting friends, family members and acquaintances is something we are all required to do daily. It is one of the easiest skills for children with autism to learn because there are few rules and the rules do not change significantly with the situation. In addition, once a child learns to say "hi," she can use the same word over and over and greet successfully. For most children, however, it is not that they cannot say "hi," it is they don't recognize when they are supposed to say it. This is where they need guidance.

✿ Practice Activities

1. Have the child greet family members daily – when the child gets up in the morning, gets home from school, when others come home from work, etc. Have the child practice responding to greetings from others. Encourage this by greeting the child in the following manner: Say "Hi (the child's name)" and wait for a response; walk closer and repeat if needed. If the child still doesn't respond, give the child a verbal prompt, "(child's name), say hi." Get other family members involved and model with each other.

2. Once the child responds to greetings from others, start to work on initiating greetings. Talk about situations in advance when greeting is needed. For example, in the car on the way to school or to visit a friend or relative, discuss and plan whom the child will greet. Role play and practice with your child while in the car and at home. Perhaps have the child exit the house or room, ring the doorbell or knock, then you answer the door and wait for her to greet you. Switch roles.

3. Ask the teacher to facilitate greeting practice at school.

4. Consider offering incentives to motivate the child to practice independently, perhaps earning a reward for greeting three times in a day.

5. Point out strangers it is OK to greet (mail carrier, police officer) and strangers who are not OK to greet (e.g., random shopper). For safety, do not allow your child to greet "random" people.

Skill 6: Join In

When you join in with others, it is polite to watch for a little while and then ask in a friendly way.

To join in with others, you:

1. Move close and smile.

2. Watch and wait for a pause.

3. Say the person's name and ask.

4. If "yes," join in. (Follow the lead of others. Do not take over the activity.)

5. If "no," do something else.

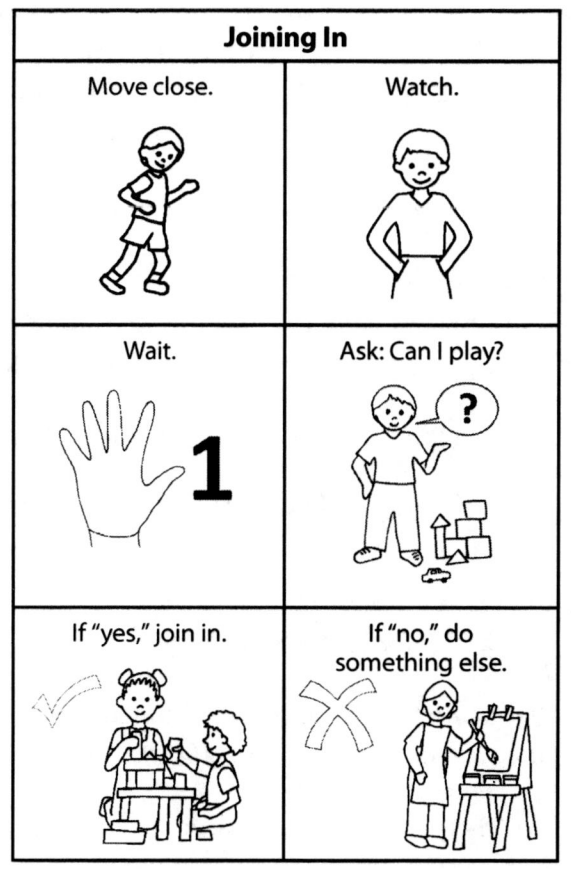

Joining In

Move close.	Watch.
Wait.	Ask: Can I play?
If "yes," join in.	If "no," do something else.

For children with autism, successfully joining in with others is especially challenging. Some children are intrusive and "butt in," taking over the activity, while more passive children struggle to move close and enter at the best opportunity. In addition to knowing the mechanics of what to say and do, correctly judging the timing is essential. Although asking is not the only way to join a group, it is one of the most direct approaches. Other options include giving encouragement to those playing, offering a suggestion for how to proceed, asking a question about what the group is doing, or entering with a greeting. These options may be suitable for those children who require an alternative to asking. The final component of this skill is learning what to do when a request to join in is turned down.

❈ Practice Activities

1. Pick a toy or game that you know your child likes. Begin to play with it. Say, "I am playing with ___." Wait for your child to ask to join you. Prompt if needed; "Say, 'Can I play'?" Do not allow the child to join in until he asks you. Make sure the child addresses you by name. Then, have him ask a sibling or friend to join in.

2. Begin an activity that you know the child likes; perhaps making cookies or popcorn or going to a favorite store. State simply what you plan to do and wait for the child to ask if he can join you.

3. Set up situations where you are having fun. Try not to give your child direct prompts. Instead, use comments. Say something like, "Hmm, I'm having fun," "Gee, this game is great," etc. Wait for the child to ask, "Can I play?" or some suitable alternative. If he cannot initiate the question, give a direct prompt ("How can you play, too?" "Say: 'Can I play?'")

4. Model joining in by asking the child if you can join him while he is engaged in an activity.

5. Set up play opportunities with 1-2 other children. Plan simple turn-taking games and activities. Prompt your child to use names and to join in as needed. Be sure to stay involved. Keep the activities and games moving quickly. Do not let your child play alone.

6. Praise your child whenever he joins in or when he responds to requests to join in.

7. Ask siblings and friends to begin favorite activities in your child's presence. Encourage your child to ask to join in.

Skill 7: Offer Encouragement

It is being kind to notice when others look upset or disappointed and then to offer encouragement.

To offer encouragement, you:

1. Smile.

2. Look at the person.

3. Call out their name.

4. Say something friendly, like, "Good try." "Keep trying." "You can do it."

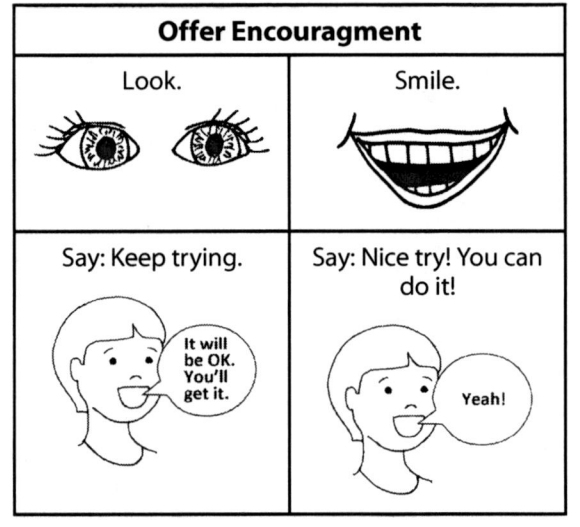

One way to help others to feel better when they are sad is to "offer encouragement." For children this is particularly relevant in situations where peers have not done as well as expected – perhaps playing a game, participating in a contest, getting a lower grade on a homework assignment or project, or making a mistake. Many children with autism are perfectionists and view mistakes or losing as "failures." We must help them to realize that it is OK to make mistakes, both for others and for themselves. Teaching them to offer encouragement to others is one way to help them.

🧩 Practice Activities

1. Set up situations where someone "fails" (gives a wrong answer, fails to catch a ball, makes a "wrong" selection). Then model offering encouragement by saying, "Good try" or "Keep trying; you can do it." Have the child repeat the words with you. Consider rewarding your child for using encouraging talk with others ("Good try.")

2. Set up relay races. They are great opportunities to cheer. Consider rewarding the person who offers the most encouragement or cheers the loudest, or even loses.

3. Use natural situations to offer encouragement – with difficult tasks, when one is losing at a game, with frustrating experiences. Prompt as necessary.

4. If your child has a tendency to boss others, set some ground rules, such as the child must offer encouragement to others in order to continue playing a game.

5. Praise your child whenever he spontaneously offers encouragement or responds when asked to offer encouragement.

6. Point out whenever you or someone else is offering encouragement.

Skill 8: Share

When you want to play with the same thing as others, when there is only one, or when there is only a small amount of something, you share.

To share, you:

1. Smile.

2. Stay calm.

3. Make a sharing plan:
    Divide something up.
    Take turns.

4. Do it.

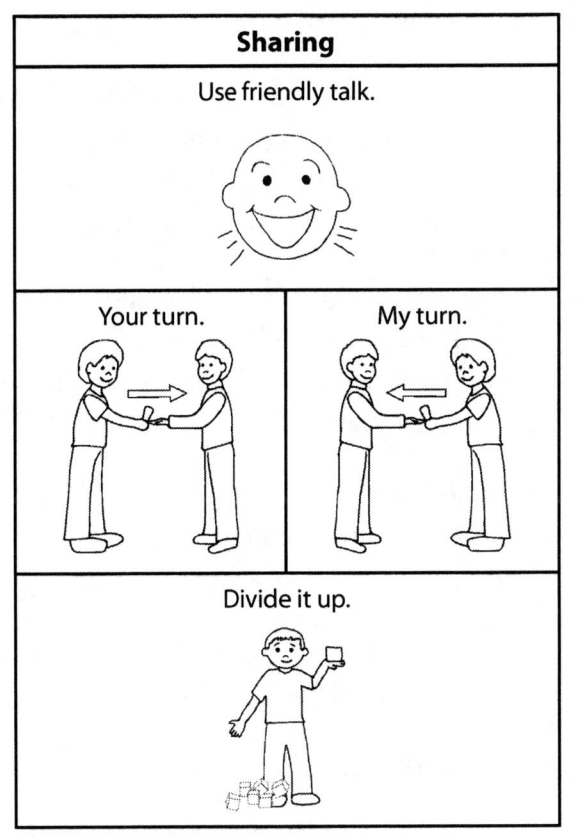

The purpose of this skill is to share with others, rather than keeping all of something for oneself. We do this by dividing something up or taking turns. An easy skill to talk about, this is difficult to learn because it requires thinking of another person, recognizing when to share in the first place, and then initiating the action. It also requires responding politely to someone when asked to share.

Set up situations and activities where your child receives an exaggerated amount of something. This helps him recognize when he can and should share with others. Your child needs help in understanding that it is courteous and polite to share with others.

✿ Practice Activities

1. Hold an entire box or carton of something your child likes. Wait until he notices and approaches you. You can (1) offer some – "I have chips. Would you like some? I'm SHARING my chips with you," or (2) wait until the child asks for some; then respond with something like "OK, I will SHARE my chips with you." (Siblings and relatives can help with this, too.)

2. Set it up in reverse. Set up situations where your child receives plenty of something, such as a bag of potato chips, carton of cookies, bag of candy, half a pizza, large box of blocks or toys, or a pile of books. Then stand next to him and wait. If he offers you some, praise for "good sharing." If he doesn't, make a comment, "Those chips sure look good." "You have ALL the chips." "I don't have ANY chips" and wait. If you don't get a response, give a direct prompt. "You have all the chips; I don't have any. Please SHARE some with me." Or you can ask a question, "You have ALL the chips. What can you do with SOME of the chips?" Try not to give your child direct prompts.

3. When your child is sharing comfortably, begin to work on saying "NO, I don't want to share with you." Set situations up similar to the above. Model how to respond when you don't want to share by saying "no" to your child when he asks for something you have. Be sure to add, "I don't want to share with you." Then have him practice the same with you.

4. Set up toys in a container or closet labeled "SHARING TOYS." These must be shared with someone else. In other words, your child may NOT play with these toys by himself; two or more must play with them together. Examples are Lego® sets, dolls or plastic characters, puppets, and costumes. Toys that belong to a specific child are labeled "NON-SHARING TOYS." They may be kept in the child's bedroom.

5. Ask the teacher to assign sharing buddies, like secret pals. During the week, each child is to share something with his buddy. At the end of the week, each child guesses who his sharing buddy was and talks about the incidents of sharing.

6. Use a "sharing table" when friends come to visit your child. Have her put toys on the table where everyone can play with them.

7. Praise your child whenever she offers to share or responds appropriately when you ask her to share.

8. Point out whenever you or someone else is sharing – strangers in public, friends, characters in books or on television, etc.

9. Talk about feeling disappointed or frustrated when someone doesn't share. When this happens, the best action is to calmly do something else.

Skill 9: Wait

Sometimes you have to wait.
When this happens you
can make a waiting plan
and do something else for a little while.

To wait, you:

1. Stay still, quiet and calm.

2. Think, "It's hard to wait, but I can do it."

3. Make a waiting plan.

4. Do it.

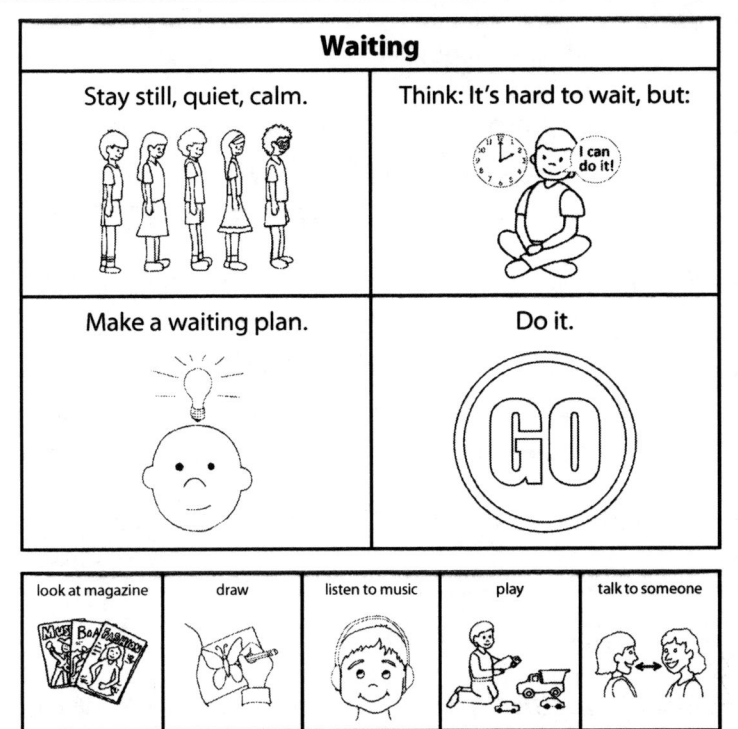

Waiting is necessary almost every day for all of us. Our children spend time waiting in lines, in traffic, for a meal, to talk to someone, to use an object, to ask for help, to be called upon in class, to use a computer, to play with a friend, and on numerous other occasions. As difficult as waiting can be, many of us find things to do to pass the time. We write, draw, listen to music, look at a magazine, talk on our phones, or talk to each other. Being able to wait appropriately is an important survival strategy, and one that is necessary for children with autism to learn.

The emphasis of this skill is on recognizing the need to wait patiently, perhaps finding something suitable to do in the meantime if the wait is lengthy. Be sure to also review when "doing something else" is not a good choice; that is, when involved in a two-way conversation (because it looks like we are not listening) or when involved in a group activity (it looks like we are not interested). Another point to discuss is when you are waiting for your child (to finish a task, get ready for school, etc.). Point out that keeping someone waiting without cause is impolite and disrespectful and why.

✿ Practice Activities

1. Games that involve taking turns, such as board games, card games, etc., are good practice activities for waiting. Emphasize who is waiting for a turn. "Doing something else" while waiting for your turn is not a good choice.

2. Look for opportunities to turn any activity into a waiting activity – waiting to talk, to change the TV channel, to order at a restaurant, to play an instrument, etc. Initially, make the turns short so there are many opportunities to practice.

3. Work with your child to develop a waiting plan. For example, while dinner is cooking, he may start homework, play a quick game, etc.

4. Talk about how people wait everyday in lines – in traffic, at school, while grocery shopping, doing chores, making dinner, etc. Waiting can give us the opportunity to "do something else," such as look at a magazine in the check-out line of the grocery store, singing to music on the radio while waiting in traffic, etc.).

5. Prompt your child to wait when necessary with "Show me waiting." Ignore protests and calmly talk your child through waiting. Praise the child frequently. Use a timer if the child has consistent difficulty waiting. Initially set it for 30 seconds or less and ask, "Show me waiting." When the timer rings, praise the child, and then set it again. Ask your child to time how long she can wait. Offer a small treat for three successes and try gradually increasing the length of the waiting time.

6. Point out whenever you or someone else is waiting and review the "waiting steps" regularly.

Skill 10: Work in a Group

Working together in a group means cooperating with others. It means finding a solution that everyone can accept. The solution may not be the one you like most.

To work in a group you:

1. Listen to the directions.

2. Keep a friendly face and voice.

3. Share your ideas and opinions.

4. Listen to others ideas and opinions.

5. Come to consensus; make a plan.

6. Stay on task and work together.

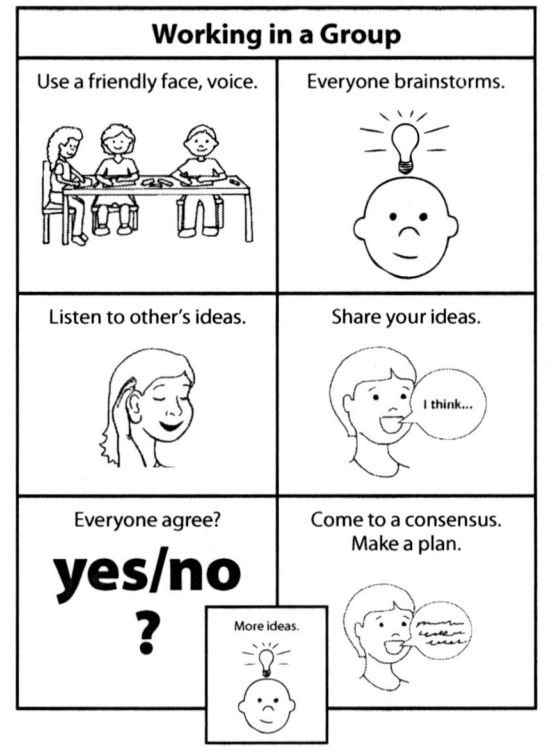

The purpose of this skill is to work with others, rather than working alone or telling others what to do. We do this by sharing our own ideas and listening to others' ideas. An easy skill to talk about, this is difficult to learn because it requires thinking of another person and recognizing when one should listen and perhaps compromise. It also requires responding to someone when asked to cooperate.

Set up situations and activities where your child must accomplish something by working with a group. Your child needs help in understanding that it is fun to cooperate with others and that it doesn't always mean "giving up" something.

✿ Practice Activities

1. Set up situations where your child must work in a group in order to receive something; for example, the group makes cookies, ice cream, or pizza, and everyone must work together to complete the task and then take part in the fun of eating. Tasks that require two or more people to complete are best.

2. Use natural situations to cooperate/work together; for example, picking up a room before leaving the house or clearing the table before dessert. Emphasize that when the group works together, the task is completed faster.

3. If your child has a tendency to be bossy, set some ground rules: "Cooperating/working in a group means listening to others' ideas and disagreeing politely if you don't like them. This means that others might disagree with your ideas, too. The idea is to come up with a plan that *everyone* can agree to."

4. Set up a "cooperation station" and place a new or different activity at the station every week. In order to engage in this activity, everyone must work together and cooperate. Choose fun activities that require more than one person to complete, such as a multi-piece puzzle, planting flowers, making a pizza from scratch, or preparing a photo collage.

5. When siblings have difficulty playing together cooperatively, start a "Cooperative Play Paper Chain." Siblings earn strips of paper (1 x 6") for demonstrating various aspects of cooperative play. They attach their individual strips to the same chain, and when the chain grows to a pre-specified number of "links," they earn a special treat or privilege, such as a pizza party or movie rental. Keep making the chain as long as possible to visually represent how well they play together. Try writing the rewards on the links as they earn them.

Teaching social skills can seem overwhelming. But with practice, you can make the lessons fun for everyone. As your child develops his repertoire of skills, you may discover that problem behaviors also resolve.

My child is nonverbal. He doesn't know how to talk. I don't think these activities apply to him. He can't participate in a discussion so how can I help him develop social skills?

In my experience, most nonverbal children with autism are capable of learning new skills and appropriate behavior. Even though you may not be able to teach your son to join in a conversation by talking, you can still focus on skills like waiting, greeting, sharing, taking turns, and cooperating, among many others. This is where your visual support tools become very important. Incorporate pictures or photos into the skills steps to show him exactly what to do. You may have to simplify the language. For example, the steps to greeting for a nonverbal child are shown in Illustration 14:1. Many augmentative communication devices such as the Dynavox Maestro™ or Attainment Company Go Talk can be programmed to speak for your child. Talk with your speech-language pathologist about the suitability of such devices for your child. In addition, establishing the now and forever social routines are also critical. Many of these do not require any language at all.

Illustration 14:1
Greetings

Smile and Wave Hello

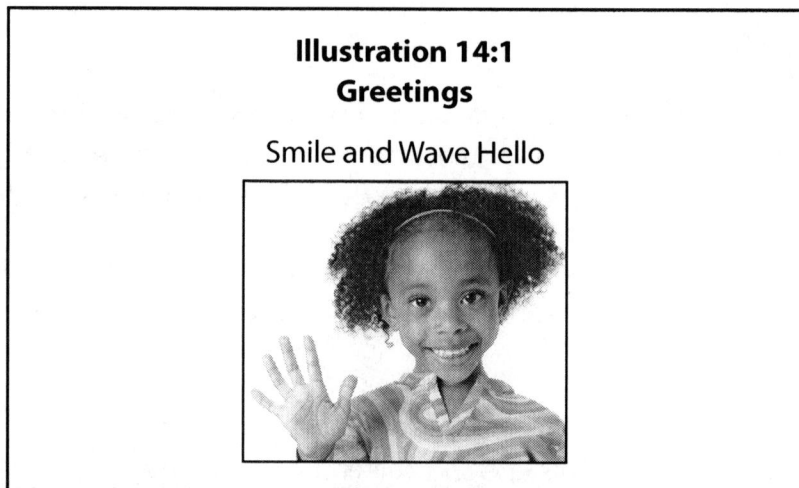

We are nearing the end of *Rules and Tools* and your toolkit is almost full. However, it is not complete without an understanding of the use of discipline and consequences as well as the potential usefulness of medication support – the subjects of our next two chapters.

Action Plan for Chapter 14: Teaching Social Skills Part II
(Select From the Choices Below)

Rules to Remember:
- ☐ Social skills require direct teaching, just like other skills.
- ☐ Teaching is everyone's job, including you.
- ☐ The context determines what skills are needed.
- ☐ Fundamental skills are integrated parts of other skills.
- ☐ Social skill deficits are one reason for challenging behavior.
- ☐ Identify specific skills for focused teaching.
- ☐ Emphasize the positive, not the negative.
- ☐ Arrange for practice activities at home.
- ☐ Arrange for practice activities in the community.
- ☐ Teach "Now and Forever" social rules.

Tools to Use:
- ☐ Social Skills Daily Practice Log
- ☐ Skill Steps
- ☐ Rewards
- ☐ Modeling
- ☐ Practice Activities

To Do:
- ☐ First skill to teach: _____
  - – Practice Activities Nos. _____
- ☐ Second skill to teach: _____
  - – Practice Activities Nos. _____
- ☐ Third skill to teach: _____
  - – Practice Activities Nos. _____

References and Further Reading

Bareket, R. (2006). *Playing it right! Social skills activities for parents and teachers of young children with autism spectrum disorders, including Asperger Syndrome and autism.* Shawnee Mission, KS: AAPC Publishing.

Benton, M., Hollis, C., Mahler, K., & Womer, A. (2112). *Destination friendship: Developing social skills for individuals with autism spectrum disorders or other social challenges.* Shawnee Mission, KS: AAPC Publishing.

Coucouvanis, J. (2005). *Super skills: A social skills group program for children with Asperger Syndrome, high-functioning autism and related challenges.* Shawnee Mission, KS: AAPC Publishing.

Jackson, N. F., Jackson, D. A., & Monroe, C. (1983). *Getting along with others: Teaching social effectiveness to children.* Champaign, IL: Research Press.

McGinnis, E., & Goldstein, A. P. (1997). *Skillstreaming the elementary school child: New strategies and perspectives for teaching prosocial skills* (rev. ed.). Champaign, IL: Research Press.

Chapter 15:
Using Consequences

Most parents anticipate a child will change her actions and behave more appropriately after being disciplined, and thereby learn to distinguish "right" from "wrong." They expect the child to learn what behavior is unacceptable by not "letting her get away with it," so maybe we lecture, scold, yell, or even spank. Perhaps we send the child to her room or to "timeout," restrict her favorite activity, or remove a privilege.

⚙ Rule: Negative consequences, when used alone, do not permanently change behavior in most children with autism.

For most typically developing children, consequence-based parenting is rather effective, and most children learn to become independently functioning adults. However, like many parents of children with autism, you have probably discovered that discipline does not permanently change your child's behavior. This is why using consequences, especially negative consequences, is presented at the end of this book, and not at the beginning. They are one of the last tools in your Parenting Toolkit to use, not the first.

What Are Consequences?

Consequences refer to the events that happen *after* a behavior. They are what maintain, strengthen, or reduce behavior, including both acceptable and unacceptable behaviors.

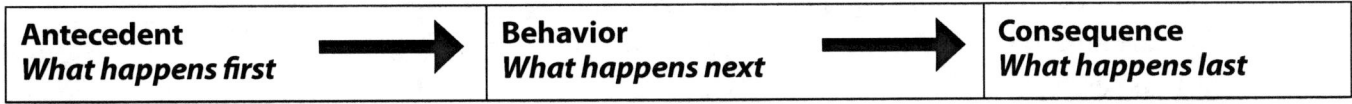

| Antecedent
What happens first | Behavior
What happens next | Consequence
What happens last |

Examples of consequences include the attention paid in response to a behavior. For example, a child shares a snack with his sibling and the parent praises him; praise is a consequence. Positive consequences, such as encouragement, feelings of satisfaction, and increased confidence, usually maintain or strengthen behaviors. In this example, the parent praises the child to encourage sharing in the future.

Another consequence is the activity, person, or object the individual either has access to or escapes from as the result of a behavior. For example, the child has homework to do and refuses to do it. Perhaps he cries and argues with the parent about doing homework. The parent sends the child to his room as a consequence. The intent of negative consequences, such as a reprimand, loss of a favorite activity, or a timeout, is to weaken or reduce the occurrence of misbehavior; however, sometimes a negative consequence actually reinforces and maintains the problem.

✿ Rule: Sometimes consequences reinforce misbehavior.

When the child who cries and argues every day about homework is disciplined by being sent to his room, he avoids the demand of homework. In reality, this consequence by the parent can maintain the behaviors of crying and whining. If the child cries loud enough and argues long enough, maybe he won't have to do any of it at all, thus escaping the task altogether. Sending him to his room allows the child to escape, so he will likely continue to whine and argue in the future when it is time for homework. A better strategy is to talk about the problem together and find out why he is resistant to homework.

If the parent talks with the child to determine the reasons why he doesn't want to do homework, she might discover the real problem, perhaps writing is extremely difficult or math problems are too complicated. Perhaps he doesn't like to leave his favorite activity. Armed with the information about the reasons for the problem, the parent can now start to problem solve more effectively.

Alternative Strategies

Assuming that sending the child to his room encourages crying and whining in the future, what can the parent do instead? Here are some ideas to try.

- ☐ Give the child three note cards with "5-minute break" written on them. Any time while doing homework he can give a card to the parent to signal that he is taking a break – until he has used all three cards. The parent sets a timer so everyone knows when each break is over. Note: The child might choose to use up all three cards at one time. That is perfectly OK.

- ☐ Sit with the child, giving him undivided attention and support.

- ☐ Place a list of phrases on the table that prompt the child with what to say when he is getting anxious and the work is hard:
  - ○ "This is hard but I will try my best."
  - ○ "I don't know how to do this. I need help please."
  - ○ "I need a break."

- ☐ "Chunk" the homework into three 20-minute sessions with 10-minute breaks in between.

- ☐ Give the child a short break after every page of homework completed.

- ☐ Write a simple story explanation and place it next to the child:
  "Sometimes my teacher gives me new work to try.
  I want to do my best work.
  I feel good when I am doing good work. That makes me happy.
  Everyone needs help learning new things. My parents will help me.
  I can try new work. I can learn how to do it."

The point is that there is a multitude of ways to intervene once you know the reason for the problem and the maintaining consequences.

⚙ Rule: Selecting consequences should be the last step of the plan, not the first.

Before using negative consequences to try to reduce or eliminate a problem behavior, you must discover the reason(s) for the problem in the first place. Usually this takes good detecting skills and lots of repeated effort. But don't despair and give up! If your plan "isn't working," review Chapters 4 and 5 to make sure you have identified all possible reasons for the problem. (There may be more than one reason!) Then consult with a professional. Finally, look at your plan and consider changing the consequences, because the consequence may inadvertently be maintaining the problem behavior. A qualified professional can help you figure this out.

The Issue of Intent: Can't Do or Won't Do?

When parents consider whether or not to discipline a child, the issue of intent plays an important role. If a child is perceived as intentionally noncompliant, disrespectful, or aggressive, we feel OK about carrying out a punishment, such as a timeout. On the other hand, if the behavior is an emotional reaction, or we suspect the child can't do a task, we are less inclined to discipline. The problem is that often we're not sure – is it a "can't do" or a "won't do" situation?

In a "can't do" situation, the child either doesn't have sufficient skills or knowledge to handle the situation or has some of the skills or knowledge but is not fluent. Remember 15-year-old Tom from Chapter 4? He had not mastered shoe tying. Negative consequences will not help the child change his behavior and learn new skills in a "can't do" situation.

In a "won't do" situation, the child has mastered the skills and is choosing not to use them. This might be the child who knows perfectly well how to take turns, but instead of waiting his turn pushes his sister off the swing at the park. In this situation, a negative consequence such as timeout, loss of the swing for the remainder of the afternoon, or removal from the park might be used as a consequence for pushing. This same child might be praised for taking turns.

Sometimes we think the problem is a "won't do" when really it is a "can't do." This is what happened to Patty, Tom's mother. Eventually, she discovered why reprimanding Tom was not helping – because reprimands did not help him learn the needed skills (shoe tying); they just made him feel bad.

When you decide to use a negative consequence, be consistent and fair. It's important for the child to know what is expected and the consequences for not following rules or infringing on the rights of others. When discipline is necessary, carry it out promptly. Be brief and to the point. Be firm but not punitive.

16-year-old Richard loved to go out to eat and to the movies with his older brother Fred when Fred was home from college on the weekends. Yet, frequently he was disruptive and even behaved dangerously in the car, making it unsafe for Fred to drive. Behavior observation indicated the misbehavior was attention seeking. Richard was excited to be in the car with his brother but couldn't safely regulate his emotions and behavior.

The family agreed that Richard was capable of riding in the car calmly and quietly. Fred made sure he had some of Richard's favorite music and picture books in his vehicle and he made a sign for the dash: "The rule is: Sit quietly and calmly." It was agreed that Fred would place three numbered sticky notes on the dash of the car marked 1, 2, and 3. As soon as Richard became disruptive, Fred removed one of the notes and said, "That's one. Please sit quietly and calmly." If Richard continued to misbehave, Fred removed the second note and said, "That's two. Please sit quietly and calmly." If Fred had to remove the third sticky note, he said, "That's three," and turned around and went home. They would then try again the next day. After a few weeks of success, new expectations were developed, and only two sticky notes were placed on the dash. A few weeks later, only one was needed.

⚙ Rule: Children with autism who learn and use skills in one environment may not automatically use them in another.

We have all heard about the children who demonstrate great behavior at home but are challenging at school, or vice versa. This is another common circumstance where "won't do" and "can't do" issues are confusing. One hallmark feature of children with autism is that they are consistently inconsistent. This is deceiving for parents and others who see or hear the child use a skill. We think, *he can do that; he does it for me,* or *I saw him do it yesterday,* and so we assume he can do it everywhere. This is a mistake! This is why each child must be taught to use new skills in multiple environments.

⚙ Rule: Negative consequences are only permissible when a child has mastered a skill or behavior in multiple environments.

We must remember that often behaviors and skills do not automatically generalize and that we have to work to teach the new rules and acceptable behavior everywhere. (Review Chapters 12-14.) Remember that it is best to teach a skill in the setting(s) where the child is likely to need it.

So, in general, you can consider using a negative consequence **in addition to positive consequences, such as rewards,** if you …

1. Know the reason for the problem (or are fairly certain)

2. Are absolutely positive that the child has mastered the skill or behavior you are asking him to do

3. And he can use the skill in multiple environments

Tool: Consequence Strategies

Guidelines for How to Respond in Ways That Won't Maintain the Problem

Redirection: Following misbehavior, the child is redirected to use the replacement behavior that everyone has agreed upon, the "new rule." This is done most often with very young children. For example, a child urinates in his pants and is redirected to urinate in the toilet; a child starts to throw and is redirected to "hands down;" a child takes a toy from another child and is redirected to another toy; a child starts to tantrum and is redirected to count to 10.

Natural Consequences: This is an event that normally or naturally occurs following a behavior if someone does not intervene to prevent it. For example, a child plays roughly with a pet and the pet scratches or bites the child; a child pushes another child and that child pushes back; a child touches a hot stove and gets burned; a child twirls objects in front of his eyes and feels calm.

Logical Consequence: This is logically related to the behavior and used when you cannot allow a natural consequence to occur. For example, a child plays with food and the food is removed for one minute; a child throws a toy and the toy is put away; a child rides his bike in the street and the bike is locked up for the rest of the day.

Withholding Reinforcement: No reinforcement is given for the behavior. For example, a child is not ready for school on time and doesn't earn a special snack in his lunch bag. A child throws a tantrum in a store and doesn't earn a special treat. A child hits a sibling at the park and loses computer time when he gets home.

Response-Cost/Loss Programs: These programs involve the loss of secondary rewards (tokens, tickets, points, etc.) in the form of a fine for misbehavior. Sometimes a loss system is called a token economy. Removing points or tokens should only occur in a "won't do" situation, when the child chooses not to follow a rule or meet an expectation, and only if he knows what to do instead.

Implementing a loss system can be risky, and I usually don't recommend it for children with autism. When some children with autism realize they are going to "lose" a ticket or token, especially one they have had to earn, they become enraged. In such cases, don't take tokens away for misbehavior. Set up the plan so that the child either earns or doesn't earn them.

Extinction: A very specific procedure that represents withholding reinforcement is extinction. In order to use it you must know the purpose of the behavior. If the purpose of a challenging behavior is to get attention, then the extinction procedure is to ignore the behavior. For example, a child who crawls under the table, a behavior that was previously reinforced by attention, is subsequently ignored until the attention-seeking behavior no longer occurs. If the purpose of the behavior is to escape or avoid a demand or a task, then the extinction procedure is to maintain the demand, thus not allowing escape or avoidance. For example, a child who crawls under the table, a behavior that was previously reinforced by avoiding the task of homework, is subsequently expected to complete homework , thus not allowing escape. Extinction is a complex procedure and extremely difficult for most adults to do consistently and correctly 100% of the time. However, it is critical that the procedure is followed every single time the identified behavior occurs in order for extinction to be successful. If the procedure is not followed every time, then the behavior is at risk of being inadvertently reinforced. Another complicating factor, called an extinction burst, is a sudden and temporary increase in the challenging behavior's frequency. In other words, behaviors often get worse before they get better. This typically occurs soon after an extinction program is initiated, and is followed by the eventual decline of the behavior targeted for elimination. For these reasons, the decision to use extinction is best made in collaboration with a qualified professional who can guide you in its use.

Examples of Loss Programs

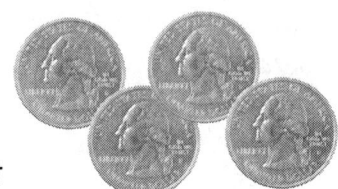

Marcus, age 16, starts each day with four quarters. Each time he swears at one of his parents, he loses a quarter. He is allowed to keep any quarters left over at the end of the day.

Matt, age 6, earns one playing card for following his morning routine, another for receiving a "good day" report from the teacher in his backpack, and two more for following directions after school and at bedtime. Each card is worth 10 minutes of electronics, but he must have four cards in order to play. He can also exchange 12 cards for a small toy. Matt loses a card for hitting, slamming doors, raising his fist, or stomping on the floor.

Franklin, age 10, uses a visual schedule of the day's activities: breakfast, get dressed, potty and teeth, car and bus, wear seatbelt, etc. He earns a star on the schedule for each activity that he transitions to and completes successfully. Each star equals a quarter. If he doesn't get a star and has an X instead, he loses one of the quarters he has earned. At the end of the day, the total number of stars and X's are counted. The number of X's is subtracted from the number of stars, and he is paid the remaining total; for example, he might have 15 stars and 5 X's, which equals 10 quarters or $2.50. If he has a "negative balance," meaning he has more X's than stars, he doesn't earn anything but doesn't "owe" anything either. He begins each day with a new start.

Parent Testimonial:

My son, Ben, was diagnosed with autism at 3 years of age. We consulted with many professionals on how to help him. We ended up going the medication route because of his eloping, aggression, ADHD, ODD, and Tourette's, when therapy alone did not help.

Something that really seemed to help him as he got old enough to understand the concept, about 6 or 7 years of age, was a reward system. He received tokens for listening and following through with directions that he was given or for having a good day with few or no bad behaviors. Immediate gratification was needed at first; for example, Dollar Store toys, snacks, DVDs, trains, or cars. Eventually, he was able to earn tokens to buy things or save them up to go somewhere. Now that he is 11, he gets his choice of immediate gratification or saving up for big things like a fish tank, etc. But he does need to physically see the tokens and/or a chart to remind him of what he is working for on a daily basis.

In the past year, he has gotten into the iPad and riding his four-wheeler. We've been able to get him to follow through by him knowing that he will lose these privileges if he doesn't follow through. I know it sounds bad to take things away, but you just need to find out what works for your child. We need him to grow and progress to become independent in the future.

We're not looking for perfection. Which one of us is perfect anyway? We want our son to manage his life one day at a time and become a decent member of society. Every day is different with my son. Every event is different even though he's been somewhere 100 times. You need to be prepared with tools that you know will move your child forward from that bad moment.

Beth Klocek

Timeout

"Timeout" means that a child is immediately isolated in a "boring" place for a few minutes after a misbehavior. The purpose is to remove adult and peer attention, or reinforcement, for misbehavior. Timeout also includes the removal of a favorite activity or the capacity to engage in a favorite activity. Sometimes timeout is called quiet time, thinking time, or cooling-down time. (Timeouts give parents a time to cool off, too!)

The decision to use timeout must be made very carefully. It is best reserved for younger children and for one or two problem behaviors that cannot be ignored, such as biting or hitting, not as a general behavior management strategy. It can be used for older children with good verbal abilities who are considered "high functioning."

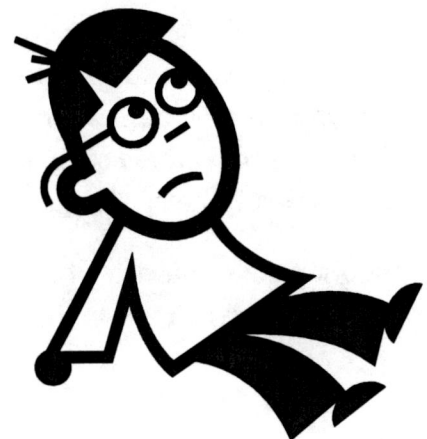

✿ Rule: Timeout works best when the child has mastered the skill or task being asked *and* he wants to be with family members and friends.

The child will more likely want to return to something that is fun and rewarding; therefore, timeout can be a very effective intervention when used as part of a comprehensive plan.

✿ Rule: Timeout should never be the only intervention.

This is because timeout does not teach your child what to do instead of the misbehavior. To learn new skills and behaviors, the child needs directed teaching and practice opportunities, as well as positive reinforcement for the desired replacement behavior. In addition, you have to know your child well when considering timeout. If your child would rather be alone, then a strategy like timeout is probably not going to be very effective because isolation is a state that your child prefers. In such cases, timeout often positively reinforces the problem behavior.

✿ Rule: When timeout is reinforcing, the child is likely to engage in the misbehavior again.

There are other instances where timeout doesn't work. For some children, timeout becomes a preferred consequence when they learn that they can escape a difficult situation or challenging task. This occurs when a child is sent to the principal's office or home when she is disruptive at school or sent to her room when she refuses to do homework. She gets to escape the demands of the classroom or of homework (or any other challenging circumstance where timeout is applied as punishment). If this happens often enough, she eventually learns to act out in order to escape. For any child, the best strategy is to find out why the child is disruptive in the first place and then address these reasons.

Place for Timeout

Timeout should be in a boring place, such as in a heavy chair with arms facing a blank wall or corner or a specific place on the floor marked by a carpet square or tape. It should not be in front of the television or in a place where your child can watch what others are doing or talk to them.

If your child cannot stay in a chair, send him to a timeout room, a place that is safe and contains no toys or valuables. It must not be a scary place, such as a small closet or a dark basement. It also cannot have furniture that he can climb or pull over onto himself. Sometimes a child's bedroom, or the end of a hallway, is a convenient and safe place for timeout. While in timeout, he may not watch television, play video games, or be on the computer. You may need to remove these activities.

Timeout places away from home can be the blank wall of a building, the floor of your vehicle, a bench at the mall, or facing a tree in the park.

Explaining Timeout

If your child is new to timeout, you must explain it to him ahead of time. A simple timeout chart is a helpful visual support. Place a photo or drawing of your child engaging in the identified problem behavior (e.g., hitting) in a square on the chart. Then draw an arrow to the next square that holds a photo of the timeout chair or place. Then place a photo of the appropriate replacement behavior (e.g., ask for help) beneath, followed by a second arrow and the reward the child is earning by asking for help.

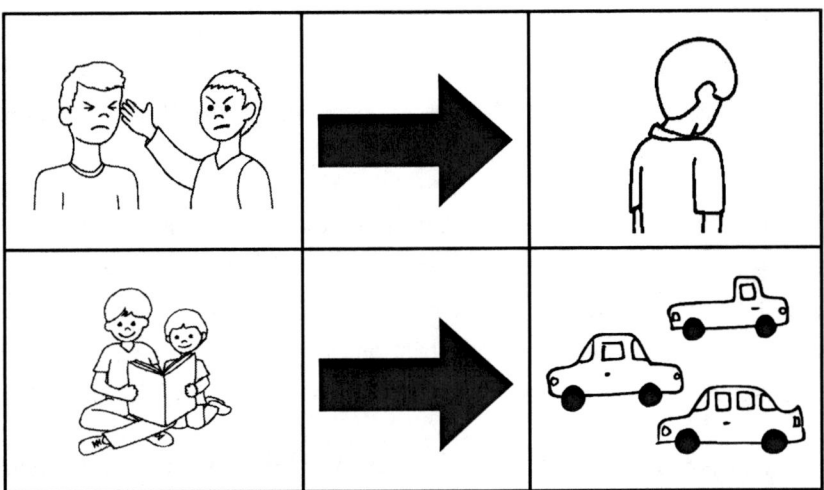

The length of timeout is usually 1 minute per year of age to a maximum of 10 minutes. For children over 2 years old, set a kitchen timer that the child can see and hear to mark the length of time (it must be placed out of reach of the child).

Practice the timeout procedure when you first introduce it, explaining each step as you walk the child through the routine. Be sure to explain the behavior for which your child will be placed in timeout, where timeout is located, and how long it lasts.

✿ Tool: Timeout Procedure

After practicing the timeout routine, you're ready to implement the procedure.

1. As soon as the target behavior occurs, name the behavior for which the child is being sent to timeout. For example, "That's biting. Timeout." Silently take the child by the wrist or direct her from behind and lead her to timeout. If needed, carry the child to the timeout area.

2. Don't engage in a power struggle with the child. Don't talk, scream, or argue. Avoid displaying anger, ignore tantrum behavior, and proceed in a calm, unemotional manner. Look straight ahead, not at your child. At this point, you are minimizing your attention to the child.

3. Calmly place the child in the timeout area and set a kitchen timer for the designated number of minutes. Record the date, behavior, and time on the Timeout Log (see page 207).

4. It is unlikely that your child will sit quietly and calmly in timeout the first few times you use it. She may cry, scream, or kick. As long as the child remains in the timeout area, ignore her. Don't tell her to stop any of these behaviors. Remember, don't look at or talk to the child while she is in timeout.

5. If your child leaves timeout, respond by quickly returning her to timeout. Be firm, yet matter-of-fact. Reset the timer. Don't argue or scold. Some very young children may need to be held in timeout temporarily to teach them to obey you. Hold the child by the shoulders from behind. Avoid eye contact and any talking. A last resort is to put the child in her bedroom with a gate in the doorway. Some parents install a ½ or ¾ door. If you don't want to block the entrance with a gate, you may hold the door shut for the 3-5 minutes of timeout or latch it from the outside. Be very careful not to leave the door locked for more than a few minutes.

6. For an older child who refuses to go to timeout, you can extend the time one minute at a time: "For every 15 seconds it takes you to get to timeout, you have 1 more minute of timeout." Then look at your watch and start counting, up to a maximum of 20 minutes. After 20 minutes is reached, and if your child has not gone to timeout, you can remove or restrict all preferred activities, such as electronics, television, outside play, snacks, etc., until he has taken the full 20 minutes of timeout that you gave him.

7. After the timer rings, say, "Timeout is finished." Lead the child back to the area where the behavior occurred or allow her to leave the timeout area when she is ready. The child may choose to stay there for a few more minutes. This is fine. Don't scold or threaten her with another timeout.

8. Treat your child normally. Some children need time to recover. I recommend waiting until the child is calm before insisting that she apologize for her behavior. It is a mistake to sit down to discuss the behavior immediately after timeout if the child is still upset because she will not be able to process what you say. It takes some children well over an hour to calm completely. Be patient.

9. If the child is still noisy when the timeout is over, I prefer to let her out of timeout, and when she is quiet, say, "Good quiet" or something similar.

10. Be sure to use timeout every time the target behavior occurs – and use it immediately. Don't threaten to use timeout or give your child a warning. When the target behavior occurs, timeout should follow immediately.

11. Make sure the child's usual environment is rewarding. Provide lots of encouragement and praise for appropriate behavior.

Timeout Log Example				
Name:			**Date:**	
Date/Time	**Place**	**Behavior (Reason for Timeout)**	**Behavior while in Timeout**	**Total Minutes**
9/6: 2:00	Play room	Bit sister in the leg when she started crying	Screaming for 5 minutes, Then cried, and was calm	10

Final Recommendations

Timeout is not easy. It requires that parents change their behavior, too. Some parents are unable to stop arguing, lecturing, or scolding. If you cannot stop this behavior in yourself, you will need to practice because timeout won't work otherwise. To increase your timeout effectiveness skills, think about the following:

1. Play with your child every day and give him lots of positive attention.

2. Be clear about the rules and your expectations. Discuss them when all of you are calm.

3. Use timeout *every time* the behavior occurs. This means you may have to use timeout multiple times a day when you start. Keep the Timeout Log to monitor your child's progress, but don't make a point to discuss it with your spouse or other relatives when your child can hear you. Instead, point out the instances of good behavior.

4. Don't threaten to use timeout; use it immediately, ideally within 10 seconds after the misbehavior. For aggressive behavior, don't give warnings. For other behaviors, you may give one warning or count to three before giving a timeout.

5. Ignore tantrums in timeout, and don't talk or lecture while your child is there.

6. Make sure that timeout is not used alone. Your plan must include positive consequences for new skills and replacement behaviors.

TIMEOUT LOG				
Name:			**Date:**	
Date/Time	**Place**	**Behavior (Reason for Timeout)**	**Behavior while in Timeout**	**Total Minutes**

Action Plan for Chapter 15: Using Consequences
(Select From the Choices Below)

Rules to Remember:
- ☐ Negative consequences, when used alone, do not permanently change behavior in most children with autism.
- ☐ Sometimes consequences reinforce misbehavior.
- ☐ Selecting consequences should be the last step of the plan, not the first.
- ☐ Children with autism who learn and use skills in one environment may not automatically use them in another.
- ☐ Negative consequences are only permissible when a child has mastered a skill or behavior in multiple environments.
- ☐ Timeout works best when a child has mastered the skill or task being asked and he wants to be with family members and friends.
- ☐ Timeout should never be the only intervention.
- ☐ When timeout is reinforcing, the child is likely to engage in the misbehavior again.

Tools to Use:
- ☐ Redirection
- ☐ Natural Consequence
- ☐ Logical Consequence
- ☐ Withholding Reinforcement
- ☐ Cost Response/Loss Program
- ☐ Timeout Procedure

To Do:
- ☐ The behavior to consequence is: _____
- ☐ The consequence is: _____

References and Further Reading

Aspy, R., & Grossman, B. G. (2012). *Designing comprehensive interventions for high-functioning individuals with autism spectrum disorders: The Ziggurat model. Textbook edition.* Shawnee Mission, KS: AAPC Publishing.

Clark, L. (1989). *The time-out solution: A parent's guide for handling everyday behavior problems.* Chicago, IL: McGraw-Hill/Contemporary Books.

Dunlap, G., Fox, L., Hemmeter, M. L., & Strain, P. (2004). *The role of time-out in a comprehensive approach for addressing challenging behaviors of preschool children.* Center on the Social and Emotional Foundations for Early Learning. Retrieved from http://csefel.vanderbilt.edu/briefs/wwb14.pdf

Forehand, R., & Long, N. (2002). *Parenting the strong-willed child: The clinically proven five-week program for parents of two- to six-year-olds.* Chicago, IL: McGraw-Hill/Contemporary Books.

Fouse, B., & Wheeler, M. (1997). *A treasure chest of behavioral strategies for individuals with autism.* Arlington, TX: Future Horizons.

Chapter 16:
Medication Support

Sometimes a child's problems are so severe that intensive behavior change programs are not sufficient, despite everyone's concentrated efforts. Sometimes a child has other problems in addition to autism, such as anxiety, hyperactivity, and difficulty attending to tasks. This is the reason for including this chapter on medication supports. Perhaps your child's behaviors are a barrier to school inclusion, an impediment to community participation, or present a physical and emotional risk to members of your family and others. Perhaps your child's pediatrician recommends medication treatment. If you are a parent of such a child, this chapter describes what you might expect. Medications are another tool for your Parenting Toolkit and can be very helpful for some children with autism.

Medications as an Additional Treatment

Medications are used to treat co-occurring conditions and specific symptoms, such as irritability, mood changes, or temper outbursts. Using medications for children with autism is controversial; education, environmental modification, and intensive behavior treatment are the preferred interventions, yet use of medication as an adjunctive therapy is increasing. Sometimes medications are used as additional treatment to reduce severe and enduring problems that are negatively impacting the child's ability to function and participate effectively in daily activities. For example, medications may help reduce the frequency or intensity of extreme or dangerous behavior in your child, such as severe self-injurious behavior, extreme aggression, persistent mood changes, excessive irritability or fear, chronic sleep disturbance, intense anxiety, severe hyperactivity, or inattention.

Medications will not eliminate these problems but may help to decrease them. Even when medication is prescribed, the child still requires intensive behavioral intervention, skill teaching, and environmental modifications. A psychiatrist once told me that when medications are effective, they have the potential to reduce a problem by 30%. If there is at least 30% improvement with medication and another 30% (or more) with behavior intervention strategies, environmental modification, and skill teaching, then at 60% or more problem reduction, we are building considerable progress!

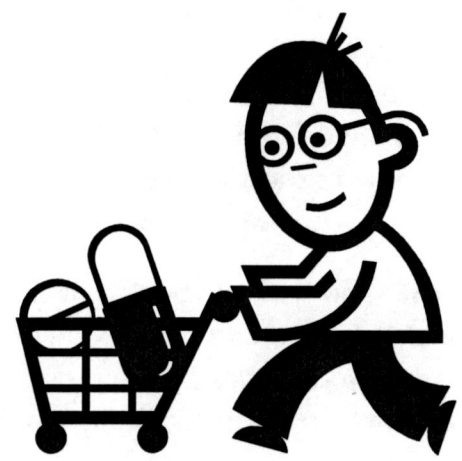

Co-Occurring Mental Health Issues and Autism

Because of language or cognitive limitations, as well as difficulty expressing and monitoring personal emotions and moods, co-occurring mental health conditions are often difficult to diagnose in persons with autism. Children are not just small adults but require special consideration. Therefore, it is wise to search out professionals who have extensive experience with autism and developmental disabilities, in addition to expertise in mental health. Such professionals include a child psychiatrist, psychologist, psychiatric nurse practitioner, or clinical social worker.

Try to find someone you like and can work with. Your local or state autism society will likely have a list of children's mental health practitioners. Not all practitioners can prescribe medications; you will need to ask if prescribing is part of their scope of practice. If not, they may work with someone who prescribes. It may also be prudent to ask how many children with autism they have seen in the past year to increase your understanding of the breadth of their experience with children with autism.

In the event you don't have a specialist in your community, try to find someone who is willing to consult with a more experienced clinician. Often major medical centers have autism and psychiatric specialty clinics with multidisciplinary teams. The specialty clinic can conduct the evaluation and make recommendations for your local practitioner.

Co-Occurring Conditions

Remember the Behavior Significance Scale presented in Chapter 3? When problems score at the "extremely significant" level, a mental health or psychiatric condition may be superimposed upon your child's autism and contribute to his unique behavior circumstances. Common conditions include the depressive disorders; attention deficit hyperactivity disorder (ADHD); anxiety disorders, including obsessive-compulsive disorder (OCD), separation anxiety disorder, and phobic disorders; and tic disorders, including Tourette syndrome. These problems are not accounted for by a diagnosis of autism. They are in addition to autism and can persist throughout a person's life, causing significant impairment to the child and additional burden to caretakers.

Autism

Mental Health Condition:
- Depression
- Anxiety
- ADHD
- OCD
- Tourette

When another condition occurs with autism, it is called a "co-occurring condition." There is mounting evidence that co-occurring conditions are a serious problem in youth with autism and can be diagnosed at very young ages. Some researchers report a higher level of mental health problems in youth with autism than in those without autism.

As a parent, your input is critical when it comes to identifying behavior changes in your child, which is essential for detecting signs and symptoms of a problem. Mental health professionals will ask you about classic signs of a problem, such as mood or appetite changes, but will also ask about unusual behaviors, such as self-injurious behavior, aggression, deterioration in language, or lack of interest in usual activities. In addition, they will ask you to share your child's family history, because often there is a biological predisposition for co-occurring conditions and sometimes a medication that is helping one family member is helpful for your child with autism.

✹ Tools: Behavior Significance Scale and Weekly Behavior Logs

> Description of the Problem
> **+**
> Behavior Changes
> Mood Changes
> Appetite Changes
> Sleep Patterns
> Unusual Behaviors
> Aggression
> Loss of Skills
> Family History
> Medical Illness
> Current Therapies,
> Treatments, and Interventions

Your child's Behavior Significance Scale and Weekly Behavior Logs (see Chapter 3) as well as any corroborating data collected by your school team or therapists can be very useful to the clinician when determining if your child has a co-occurring condition or complex behavior challenges. Be sure to ask your child's teacher if she has collected any data on the problem. The specialist will ask for information about the frequency, intensity, duration of the problem, and any exacerbating factors, such as illness, setting, time of day, or recurring event. This information will also help determine if medication has a reasonable chance of helping. If you and your team have not been collecting data on the problems using one of these tools, it would be wise to start. Then you and your team will have the most valuable baseline information and current data for to share with your child's clinician, and you will have the necessary facts to evaluate your child's progress during and after treatment.

The clinician will review your child's response to behavioral interventions with you. If you have never tried any behavioral interventions or environmental modifications, medication is probably not the best first choice. In most cases, medication is considered a supportive intervention, not a front-line treatment.

⚙ Rule: Medication is a supportive treatment in autism, not a primary treatment.

If your child is diagnosed with a co-occurring condition, such as OCD or ADHD, specific treatment for the condition is possible, and intervention may improve quality of life for your entire family. The clinician will discuss a variety of options with you, including medication if there is a reasonable chance that the problem will respond favorably to treatment. Ultimately, it is your decision as a parent to consent to a medication trial. Such a decision is not to be taken lightly because all medications have the potential for adverse, or negative effects, in addition to the potential to help. You must weigh the risk of side effects against the potential benefit of treatment.

To Treat or Not to Treat With Medications

The decision to use medications to help your child is a serious one, and one that clinicians and parents must make together. When successful, medications can reduce symptoms, such as extreme agitation, irritability, temper outbursts, repetitive behaviors, anxiety, fears, or depressed mood. Some medications can help to reduce extreme hyperactivity and poor impulse control. Others are used to help sleep, compulsions, tics, or seizures.

When a clinician suggests a medication for your child, it is essential to identify the specific problem or symptom to be treated and to quantify the degree to which it interferes with daily functioning. The Behavior Significance Scale can help you decide this.

Treat with medications when:

1. Education, environmental modification, and intensive behavior treatment have failed to sufficiently reduce the problem.

2. Your child's behaviors are a barrier to school inclusion, an impediment to community participation, or present a physical and emotional risk to members of your family and others.

3. A co-occurring condition has been diagnosed by a qualified mental health professional and there is a reasonable chance that the problem will respond favorably to medication treatment.

Do *not* treat with medications when:

1. Trying to improve a bad environment (such as an unsuitable or inappropriate setting where help and support for the child are minimal or absent). You need to institute environmental modifications first.

2. There is no emergency, and you have time to consider all options, including no treatment.

3. You and your spouse disagree about using medication; more thoughtful discussion is needed.

4. You have not tried the problem-solving and skill-building tools and strategies presented in Chapters 1-15 of this book.

5. When other treatment options supported by clinical research have not been tried.

6. The clinician cannot give you a specific reason for prescribing medication.

Information Needed by the Prescriber

In addition to details about the problem, including your data from home and school, your child's clinician will need complete information about your child's health status in order to be able to choose the right medication and dose. This includes your child's:

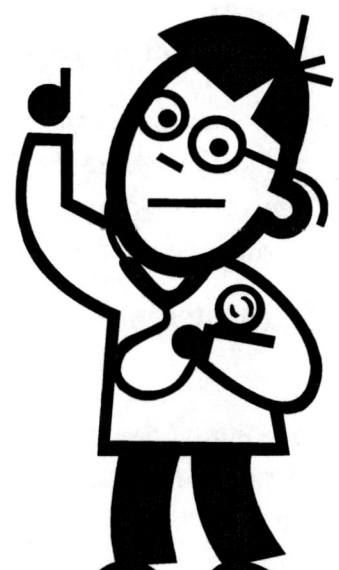

- Medical history

- Conventional medications (names, dose, and frequency)

- Herbal or alternative remedies (names, dose, and frequency)

- Vitamin therapy (names, dose, and frequency)

- Nutritional supplements

This information is necessary to discover any contraindication to specific medications and to determine potential interactions or effects that might pose a safety risk for your child. For example, some supplements can reduce the effectiveness of a medication by altering the amount of medication in a child's body. Others can enhance absorption of the medication. Bring the prescription and non-prescription bottles with you if you don't have time to write this information down.

Tell the clinician if your child cannot swallow tablets; this will limit the medication options as not all medications come in liquid form or can be crushed or dissolved, especially extended-release formulations. In the meantime, you may want to start to teach your child to swallow small tablets. Practice with tiny candies, such as mini-M&Ms or Tic Tacs.

⚙ Rule: Gather as much information about the medication as you can.

As a parent, you will be asked to sign informed consent to the medication. This will become a part of your child's medical record. Don't be afraid to ask specific questions about the medication and how it is expected to help your child. Questions might include:

- What is the target symptom(s) in my child that the medicine is expected to treat?

- What behavior change can I expect to see if the medicine is doing what it is supposed to?

- How long before I can expect to see results?

- Will my child need baseline laboratory studies, any other tests, or periodic monitoring?

- What are the potential side effects and how should I manage them?

- How long can I expect my child to be on this medication?

- Who can I call if I have further questions or concerns?

⚙ Rule: Change one intervention approach at a time.

When a new medication is introduced, it is wise to keep your behavior intervention plan and environmental modifications the same for at least a month. If you introduce a new behavior plan at the same time you start a new medication, you won't know if any improvement (or problem) is because of the medication or the behavior plan. Change one intervention at a time while continuing data collection on the Weekly Logs.

⚙ Tool: Medication Effect Checklist

Usually a system to monitor the chosen target behavior as well as any adverse events is developed. The Medication Effect Checklist (see page 219) can help you and your child's clinician review the effects of the medication prescribed. Complete it before your child takes the first dose of medicine. In addition to your other logs, this checklist is the baseline against which you can measure any medication changes, including negative effects. Then, prior to each return visit, complete another copy and take it with you to the appointment.

⚙ Rule: Response to medications is often different for children with autism than for typically developing children.

All medications have the potential for negative side effects. With some medications, children with autism appear to be more susceptible to adverse effects than typically developing children. Remember, each child is different, which often means finding a medication that is effective, with few side effects, takes some trial and error.

The Medication Effect Checklist can help you formulate the right questions to ask the child's clinician and help you address your concerns. The clinician may wish to copy your completed form(s). If so, be sure to keep copies for yourself. That way you too can review your child's progress over time. Keep the forms in a notebook or three-ring binder for easy access.

Once a medication is started, communicate any concerns you have to your child's clinician. Some medications should not be stopped abruptly, depending upon the dose; therefore, check with the clinician before stopping a medicine. Report any new or unusual behaviors immediately. As a parent, you are likely the first person to notice any adverse effects. Be aware that they may be due to the medication, and not some other reason.

Medications

Many of the medications that are typically used are considered "off label." That is, the Federal Drug Administration (FDA) has not approved the drug's use in children (frequently because the formal application process and necessary studies required by the FDA is costly). Even so, there is often extensive medical literature to support off-label use.

Hyperactivity, Inattention, and Poor Impulse Control

Some of the medications used to treat hyperactivity, inattention, oppositionality, poor impulse control, and explosive rage are called stimulants. They include methylphenidate (Ritalin, Concerta, Metadate, Methylin), dextroamphetamine (Dexedrine, Dextrostat), dexmethylphenidate (Focalin), and amphetamine/dextroamphetamine (Adderall). When using these medications, a typical concern is loss of appetite and weight loss. The clinician will monitor your child's weight. To help your child maintain her weight, consider the following modifications to your child's diet.

Maintaining Weight

☐ A big breakfast, one that includes a protein (meat, eggs, cheese, yogurt, protein shake), before taking the medication if possible.

☐ "Dinner foods" for breakfast, such as pasta, chicken, breakfast pizza.

☐ Energy or granola bars for lunch if your child doesn't eat the school lunch.

☐ Saving your child's dinner for later in the evening, especially if he doesn't eat at dinnertime but is hungry later.

☐ A snack pre-prepared in the refrigerator (plate of cheese and crackers, fresh fruit, yogurt) or in her room, if your child gets out of bed during the night because she is hungry.

Other adverse effects of stimulants include increased agitation and irritability, unusual muscle movements or other tics, and sleep disturbance. If your child has difficulty settling for sleep, you may have to give the medicine earlier in the day. Sometimes another medication is added to help your child settle at night. In some youth with autism, their obsessions worsen as focus increases (even for those things they like to do). Be sure and discuss these and any other concerns with your child's clinician.

Non-stimulant medications used to treat the same behaviors include atomoxetine (Strattera), guanfacine (Tenex), and clonidine (Catapres), which are discussed later.

Irritability, Temper Outbursts, and Aggression

Atypical antipsychotic agents, sometimes called new or second-generation antipsychotics, have become increasingly popular since the FDA approved risperidone (Risperdal) and aripiprazole (Abilify) for the treatment of irritability in children and teens with autism. Risperidone has been found effective in decreasing severe tantrums, aggression, and self-injurious behavior. Aripiprazole is used to treat similar behaviors. Other examples of atypical antipsychotic medications are ziprasidone (Geodon), quetiapine (Seroquel), olanzapine (Zyprexa), asenapine (Saphris), Paliperidone (Invega), and clozapine (Clozaril). Older, typical antipsychotics including haloperidol (Haldol) are also still used to treat severe aggression.

Sleepiness is a common side effect of these medications. Therefore, the medication is typically started at night. Usually after 4-8 weeks, a child adapts to the sedative effects, and doses may be given during the day. Any unusual, involuntary movements, such as facial grimacing, muscle twitching, or jerking, should be reported immediately as they likely mean that the medication should be discontinued.

Severely increased appetite and subsequent weight gain are a concern with some of these medications. If a child experiences increased appetite, weight gain does not typically diminish with time. Therefore, some children may become markedly overweight unless we work to help them. It is extremely important to monitor your child's weight. In addition, you will likely have to modify your child's diet.

Dietary Modifications

☐ Replace sugar-containing drinks with water.

☐ Dilute fruit juice with water or sparkling water.

☐ Replace soft drinks with sparkling water mixed with a small amount of juice.

☐ Increase intake of fresh fruits, vegetables, and fiber.

☐ Choose low-fat products.

☐ Reduce carbohydrates, such as potatoes, pasta, pizza, bread, and sugared cereals.

☐ Monitor serving sizes and portions, especially for chips and other snacks.

☐ Prepare snacks in advance by portioning small amounts into small zip-lock bags.

☐ Reduce and preferably eliminate sugared candy and treats, such as cookies and cakes.

Other life style modifications include increasing exercise. Some ideas to consider include the following:

Exercise Plan

• Walking	• Shooting baskets
• Bike riding	• Kicking a ball
• Chase game	• Running
• Dancing	• Gymnastics
• Hiking	• Reduced time in sedentary activities
• Swimming	• House chores
• Cycling	

Although less well studied than some antipsychotics, other medications used to treat irritability and aggression include trazodone (Desyrel) and N-acetyl-cysteine (NAC).

Depression, Anxiety, and Obsessions

Selective serotonin reuptake inhibitors (SSRI) are one of the many classes of antidepressants. They include fluoxetine (Prozac), paroxetine (Paxil), citalopram (Celexa), escitalopram (Lexapro), sertraline (Zoloft), and fluvoxamine (Luvox). Some of the SSRIs are approved by the FDA to treat OCD or depression in children and teens.

Children and teens with autism may be more susceptible to side effects of SSRIs than typically developing children. One such adverse effect is activation. "Activation" means increased excitability, hyperactivity, moodiness, agitation, or silliness. Because of these concerns, SSRI dosages are increased in children with autism very slowly; therefore, it may take up to 8-10 weeks to achieve moderate total daily doses. The clinician will monitor your child very closely when an SSRI is initiated and whenever the medication dosage is increased.

Other common side effects of SSRIs include nausea, sometimes vomiting, and sedation. Finally, SSRIs carry a FDA "black box" warning for increased suicidal thinking and behavior. If you are concerned about any of these events, contact your clinician.

Sleep Disorders and Tics

The alpha-2-agonists, guanfacine (Tenex and Intuniv) and clonidine (Catapres), are used to treat ADHD, sleep problems, tic disorders, agitation, and aggression. These medications have the potential to lower blood pressure and can be sedating. Children may also experience constipation, dry mouth, and mid-sleep awakening. The clinician will likely take your child's blood pressure at follow-up appointments. Melatonin is a natural hormone that is sometimes used to induce sleep with minimal risk for daytime sedation or other side effects.

Seizures and Mood Problems

The anti-epileptics (AEDs) are used to stabilize mood in addition to treating seizures. Many are available, and all work differently with varying side effects. Sometimes AEDs are used in combination with other medications to help them work more effectively. AEDs include valproate, valproic acid (Depakote, Depakene), lamotrigine (Lamictal), carbemazepine (Tegretol), oxcarbazepine (Trileptal), topiramate (Topamax), and gabapentin (Neurontin). Most of these medications require regular blood draws to monitor blood levels. Some have drug interactions. Others can cause bruising, rash, weight gain, or sedation. Topiramate, as well as N-acetyl-cysteine, are occasionally used to treat skin picking.

The use of medications in children with autism is on the rise. Some medications are undergoing rigorous study, yet most are still considered experimental. Your decision to use medications must weigh the risks of side effects versus the benefits of treatment. If you decide to use medications, educate yourself about the reason for the medication, familiarize yourself with brand and generic names, and be aware of adverse effects. Monitor your child carefully, especially when a drug is first started. Discuss any concerns with your child's clinician, and remember medication is not a miracle cure. *Medline Plus,* developed by the National Library of Medicine, provides information to help you discuss medications, ask the right questions, and make the best decisions with your healthcare provider. It is available at http://www. nlm.nih.gov/medlineplus/druginformation.html

Remember, medication alone is not an effective plan. Your child also requires intensive behavioral intervention, skill teaching, and environmental modifications.

Action Plan for Chapter 16: Medication Support
(Select From the Choices Below)

Rules to Remember:
- [ ] **Medication is a supportive treatment in autism, not a primary treatment.**
- [ ] **Gather as much information about the medication as you can.**
- [ ] **Change one intervention approach at a time.**
- [ ] **Response to medications is often different for children with autism than for typically developing children.**

Tools to Use:
- [ ] **Behavior Significance Scale**
- [ ] **Weekly Behavior Log**
- [ ] **Medication Effect Checklist**

To Do:
- [ ] **Name of medication:** _____
- [ ] **Reason for medication:** _____
- [ ] **Monitoring plan:** _____

MEDICATION EFFECT CHECKLIST

Child's Name: _____   Date: _____

Clinician's Name and Telephone Number: _____

Name(s) of Medication and Dose(s):

Reason for Medication:

Weight: _____lbs. ☐ Increase ☐ Decrease ☐ No change

Appetite: ☐ Increase ☐ Decrease ☐ No change **Thirst:** ☐ Increase ☐ Decrease ☐ No change

---

Physical Symptoms: ☐ Nausea/vomiting ☐ Rash ☐ Dizziness ☐ Stomach pain ☐ Headache
☐ Blurred vision ☐ Tremor ☐ Drooling ☐ Dry mouth ☐ Bruising ☐ Other pain ☐ Picking at skin
☐ Tics/unusual movements ☐ Change in urine habits ☐ Change in bowel habits

---

Nightly Sleep: _____ hours ☐ Increase ☐ Decrease ☐ No change
☐ Difficulty settling ☐ Difficulty awakening ☐ Difficulty remaining asleep ☐ Early awakening
☐ Nightmares ☐ Daytime drowsiness ☐ Napping ☐ No change

Attention Span: ☐ Increase ☐ Decrease ☐ No change

Focus/Concentration: ☐ Increase ☐ Decrease ☐ No change

Activity Level: ☐ Increase ☐ Decrease ☐ No change

Energy Level: ☐ Increase ☐ Decrease ☐ No change

Impulse Control: ☐ Increase ☐ Decrease ☐ No change

Mood Swings: ☐ Increase ☐ Decrease ☐ No change

Temper Outbursts: ☐ Increase ☐ Decrease ☐ No change

Irritability: ☐ Increase ☐ Decrease ☐ No change

Aggression: ☐ Increase ☐ Decrease ☐ No change

Sadness: ☐ Increase ☐ Decrease ☐ No change

Anxieties/Worries: ☐ Increase ☐ Decrease ☐ No change

Suicidal Thoughts/Behavior: ☐ Increase ☐ Decrease ☐ No change

---

Social Withdrawal: ☐ Increase ☐ Decrease ☐ No change

Happiness: ☐ Increase ☐ Decrease ☐ No change

Calm: ☐ Increase ☐ Decrease ☐ No change

Other Comments/Concerns/Questions:

References and Further Reading

Correll, C. (2008). Antipsychotic use in children and adolescents: Minimizing adverse effects to maximize outcomes. *Journal of the American Academy of Child & Adolescent Psychiatry, 47*(1), 9-20.

Coucouvanis, J., Hallas, D., & Farley, J. (2012). Autism spectrum disorder. In E. L. Yearwood, G. S. Pearson, & J. A. Newland (Eds.), *Child and adolescent behavioral health: A resource for advanced practice psychiatric and primary care practitioners in nursing* (pp. 238-261). Cambridge, UK: Wiley-Blackwell.

Coury, D. L., Anagnostou, E., Manning-Courtney, P., Reynolds, A., Cole, L., McCoy, R., Whitaker, A., & Perrin, J. M. (2012). Use of psychotropic medication in children and adolescents with autism spectrum disorders. *Pediatrics, 130*(2), S69-S76.

Douglas-Hall P., Curran S., Bird V., & Taylor D. (2011). Aripiprazole: A review of its use in the treatment of irritability associated with autistic disorder patients aged 6-17. *Journal of Central Nervous System Disorders, 3*, 143-153.

Findling, R. L. (2005). Pharmacologic treatment of behavioral symptoms in autism and pervasive developmental disorders. *The Journal of Clinical Psychiatry, 66* (Supp l10), 26-31.

Joshi, G., Petty, C., Wozniak, J., Henin, A., Fried, R., Galdo, M., & Biederman, J. (2010). The heavy burden of psychiatric comorbidity in youth with autism spectrum disorders. A large comparative study of a psychiatrically referred population. *Journal of Autism and Developmental Disorders, 40*(11), 1361-1370.

Leyfer, O., Folstein, S., Bacalman, S., Davis, N., Dinh, E., Morgan, J., & Lainhart, J. (2006). Co-morbid psychiatric disorders in children with autism: Interview development and rates of disorders. *Journal of Autism and Developmental Disorders, 36*(7), 849-861.

Liu, X., Hubbard, J. A., Fabes, R. A., & Adams, J. B. (2006). Sleep disturbances and correlates of children with autism spectrum disorders. *Child Psychiatry and Human Development, 37*(2), 179-191.

Matson J. L., & Goldin, R. L. (2013). Comorbidity and autism: Trends, topics and future directions. *Research in Autism Spectrum Disorders, 7*(10), 1228-1233.

McCracken, J. (2005). Safety issues with drug therapies for autism spectrum disorders, *Journal of Clinical Psychiatry, 66*(10), 32-37.

McDougle, C. J., Scahill, L., Aman, M. G., McCracken, J. T., Tierney, E., Davies, M., Eugene, A. L., Posey, D. J., Martin, A., Ghuman, J. K., Shah, B., Chuang, S. Z., Swiezy, N. B., Gonzalez, N. M., Hollway, J., Koenig, K., McGough, J. J., Ritz, L., & Vitiello, B. (2005). Risperidone for the core symptom domains of autism: Results from the study by the autism network of the research units on pediatric psychopharmacology. *The American Journal of Psychiatry, 162*(6), 1142-1148.

Meyers, S. M., Johnson, C. P., & the Council on Children with Disabilities. (2007). Management of children with autism spectrum disorder. *Pediatrics, 120*, 1160-1182. Retrieved from http://www.pediatrics.org/cgi/content/full/120/5/1162

NYU Langone Medical Center (n.d.). *Pill swallowing made easy.* Retrieved from http//www.aboutourkids. org/articles/pill_swallowing_made_easy

Oswald, D. P., & Sonenklar, N. A. (2007). Medication use among children with autism spectrum disorders. *Journal of Child and Adolescent Psychopharmacology, 17*(3), 348-355.

Rains, A., & Scahill, L. (2006). Nonstimulant medications for the treatment of ADHD. Journal of Child and Adolescent Psychiatric Nursing, *19*(1), 44-47.

Santosh, P. J., Baird, G., Pityaratstian, N., Tavare, E., & Gringras, P. (2006). Impact of comorbid autism spectrum disorders on stimulant response in children with attention deficit hyperactivity disorder: A retrospective and prospective effectiveness study. *Child: Care, Health and Development, 32*(5), 575-583.

Scahill, L., Koenig, K., Carroll, D., & Pachler, M. (2007). Risperidone approved for the treatment of serious behavioral problems in children with autism. *Journal of Child and Adolescent Psychiatric Nursing, 20*(3), 188-190.

Scahill, L., & Pachler, M. (2007). Treatment of hyperactivity in children with pervasive developmental disorders. *Journal of Child and Adolescent Psychiatric Nursing, 20*(1), 59-61.

Tsai, L. Y. (2001). *Taking the mystery out of medications in autism/Asperger Syndrome: A guide for parents and non-medical professionals.* Arlington, TX: Future Horizons.

Williams, K., Wheeler, D. M., Silove, N., & Hazell, P. (2010). Selective serotonin reuptake inhibitors (SSRIs) for autism spectrum disorders (ASD). *Cochrane Database of Systematic Reviews, 8,* CD004677. doi:10.1002/14651858.CD004677.pub2

Chapter 17:

The Final Chapter: Putting It All Together

Congratulations! You are almost at the end of *Rules and Tools* and well on the way to finalizing your own plan. The remaining tool for your Parenting Toolkit is the Master Action Plan (MAP) detailed in Illustration 17:1. The MAP summarizes your Action Plans from all of the previous chapters and guides your personal planning in the future. Let's return to Sam and his Weekly Behavior Log that you first reviewed in Chapter 3. Sam's log illustrates problems with tantrums. His Master Action Plan looks like this.

Illustration 17:1
Sam's Master Action Plan

Problem Description

1. Problem behavior: *Tantrums (crying, screaming, sometimes hitting)*

2. Rule of 5: Will the problem matter in five weeks, five months, or five years? (Yes)/No

   Why or why not? *May worsen as he ages; needs to learn self control, handle "no"*

3. When is the problem most and least likely to occur?

   Most: *When he has to leave park/pool, loses a game, not his turn, told "no"*

   Least: *When we use a timer*

4. Where is the problem most and least likely to occur?

   Most: *Favorite places like Grandma's, park, pool, at home*

   Least: *Camp*

5. With whom is the problem most and least likely to occur?

   Most: *Parents, Grandparents*

   Least: *Camp counselors*

6. The significance of the problem is ☐Mild ☐Moderate ☒ Severe ☐Extreme

7. The reasons for the problem include: *To protest when he can't have something, a transition when he has to stop something he likes, an unexpected event, anxiety when he is not prepared, his need to win and be first, misinterpreting the event, unknown expectations*

8. The possible antecedents for this problem are: ☐ Environment ☐Sensory ☒Communication ☐Physical/Biological ☒ Required Skills/Required Knowledge

---

Interventions

1. Antecedent modifications might include: *More use of the timer, giving warnings*

2. What exactly do I want the child to do instead of the problem behavior? *Transition between activities without screaming, stay calm, handle "no," share, be a good sport*

3. The replacement behavior(s), new rule(s), new skill(s), or new routine(s) to be practiced and reinforced are:

    ☐ *Staying calm when transitioning from the park, pool, Grandma's*

    ☐ *Staying calm when it is not his turn to choose*

    ☐ *Staying calm when told "no"*

4. The type of reward program is:

    ☐ Primary rewards

    The menu of rewards will include: (include the amount of reward)

    ○ _____

    ○ _____

    ○ _____

    ☒ Secondary rewards are: *Tokens on a strip* that will be exchanged for:

    ○ *Extra story at bedtime (3 tokens)* _____

    ○ *Ice cream at bedtime (5 tokens)* _____

    ○ *Extra trip to the park/Grandma's on Saturday (10 tokens)* _____

    ○ *Trip to the Dollar Store (20 tokens)* _____

5. The schedule of reinforcement is: *Continuous* _____

6. The communication plan includes:

    ☒ Visual schedule: *Of each day and whose turn to choose an activity*

    ☒ Visual support/Tool(s)

    ○ *Timer when getting ready to leave* _____

    ○ *First/Then chart in public* _____

    ○ *Calming routine* _____

    ☒ Verbal strategies

    ○ *Prompt before unacceptable behavior with "quiet voice," or calm hands* _____

    ○ *Extra praise and encouragement for attempts to stay calm* _____

    ○ _____

7. The consequences for the problem behavior will be:

☒ Redirection	☐ Natural consequences
☐ Logical consequence	☒ Withholding reinforcement: *Loses computer if hits at camp*
☐ Loss program	☐ Timeout
☐ None at this time	☐ Other

8. Medication supports are:

    ☐ None

    ☒ *Methylphenidate for attention and focus problems, melatonin for sleep*

9. Ongoing data collection and monitoring of the plan will occur on the:

☐ Daily Behavior Log	☐ Problem Behavior Record
☒ Weekly Behavior Log	☐ Behavior Information Tool
☐ Behavior Significance Scale	☐ Sleep Chart
☒ Medication Effect Checklist	☐ Other

Teaching New Skills and Routines

1. One new/unexpected/stressful situation for my child is: *Trying on shoes at the mall*

    The preparation plan will include:

    ☒ Getting Ready Checklist

    ☒ Priming for "What If?"

    ☒ Other: *Practice shoe store at home, Store Rules*

2. One "Now and Forever" skill/task/routine to teach my child is: *Make his bed*

    All of the following are prepared and ready to use to teach:

    ☒ The task analysis (write out the steps of the task)

    ☒ Decision: Backward/forward chain?

    ☒ Reward system:

        ☐ Primary rewards

        The menu of rewards will include: (include the amount of reward)

          ○ _____

          ○ _____

          ○ _____

☒ Secondary rewards are: *Tokens on a strip* that will be exchanged for:

- ○ *Extra story at bedtime (3 tokens)*
- ○ *Ice cream at bedtime (5 tokens)*
- ○ *Extra trip to the park/Grandma's on Saturday (10 tokens)*
- ○ *Trip to the Dollar Store (20 tokens)*

☒ Visual tool(s).

- ○ *Photos of each step on a poster by his bed*
- ○ _____

☒ Materials: *Bed linens, pillow*

☒ Setting: *Bedroom*

☒ Context: link between skill and need to teach it: *Maintain organization*

☒ Time: *Every morning before breakfast*

☒ People who will teach: *Mom on weekdays, Dad on weekends*

☒ Directions: clear steps in visual format: *See photos in bedroom*

☒ Method to monitor success and problems. *Chart on the bedroom wall*

3. A detailed master schedule for daily routines is written and agreed upon. (Yes)/No

4. The 1-3 social skills to focus teaching will be:

☐ Ask for help	☐ Ask a question on the topic
☒ Be a good sport	☐ Give and receive compliments
☐ Greet (beginner/intermediate)	☐ Join in
☐ Offer encouragement	☒ Share
☐ Wait	☐ Work in a group
☐ Other _____	☐ Other _____

5. The teaching plan will include:

☒ Social Skills Daily Practice Log

☒ Skills Steps

☐ Reward system:

- ☐ Primary rewards

  The menu of rewards will include: (include the amount of reward)

  - ○ _____
  - ○ _____
  - ○ _____

☒ Secondary rewards are: *Tokens on a strip* _____ that will be exchanged for:

    ○ *Extra story at bedtime (3 tokens)* _____

    ○ *Ice cream at bedtime (5 tokens)* _____

    ○ *Extra trip to the park/Grandma's on Saturday (10 tokens)* _____

    ○ *Trip to the Dollar Store (20 tokens)* _____

☒ Visual tool(s)

    ○ *Super Skills chart for Sharing* _____

    ○ *Super Skills chart for Being a Good Sport* _____

    ○ _____

☒ Materials: *Board games, outdoor games, sharing toys* _____

☒ Settings: *Home, Grandma's house, camp* _____

☒ Context: link between skill and need to teach it: *Builds friendships, ability to get along with others*

☒ Time: When *daily at camp and every evening at home* _____

☒ People who will teach: *Parents, family members, counselors* _____

☒ Practice activities will include:

○ *Sharing table* _____

○ *Designated box of sharing toys at home* _____

○ *Board game every night* _____

Sam's Master Action Plan illustrates how some of the same visual supports and reinforcements can be used for both managing problem behavior and teaching new skills. In this way several concerns can be addressed at the same time. In other words, multiple individual plans are not needed, but his plan is especially helpful when trying to communicate the focus of intervention to others. The MAP can be shared with other family members, such as grandparents, as well as teachers and counselors, sitters, and therapists. Now everyone can be on the same page. Armed with your MAP, you and your team are ready to begin the process of behavior change. However, there are still a few more things to consider. One is how to tell whether or not the plan is working.

Monitoring Ongoing Progress

Once you implement your plan, it is a good idea to continue collecting data to help you determine the plan's effectiveness. Choose from the many tools in this book, such as the Daily or Weekly Log, Sleep Chart, Social Skill Daily Practice Log, or the Behavior Information Tool. All of these tools are described in Chapter 4.

The data tell you whether or not your methods are working. Look for an increase in the frequency of desired behavior and note when it occurs, such as transitioning to bedtime, asking for help with homework, or sharing with siblings. Even when you don't see a decrease in the frequency of problem behavior such as yelling or hitting, your plan is working if your child is demonstrating a higher frequency of appropriate behavior than previously. First, your child has to learn the skills, then he can start to apply them.

Completing the Behavior Significance Scale (Chapter 3) at the end of each week can also indicate if the duration or intensity of the problem behavior is decreasing, even if the frequency is not. Note the settings where the problem behavior continues to occur. You may notice that behavior is better in a few situations, even though not all situations. Look at what is happening and compare problem situations with those that are improving. Notice what you are doing differently, if anything. A positive change in any direction is a good sign and means you should continue your plan.

If you see no increase in positive behavior or decrease in problem behavior at all after a week or two, just hold tight and follow your plan. If you are still concerned, be sure to consult with a professional.

How Long Before You Will See Results?

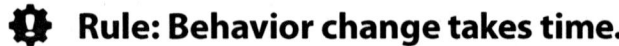 **Rule: Behavior change takes time.**

An interesting study by Lally and colleagues (2010) revealed that when adults want to develop a relatively simple habit, like eating a piece of fruit every day or taking a 10-minute walk, it could take over two months of daily repetitions before the behavior becomes a habit. However, there was marked variation in how long habits took to form, anywhere from 18 days to 254 days in the habits examined in the study with an average of 66 days. So, although that study did not talk about children with autism, the results tell us that developing an automatic habit, meaning a behavioral response, can take a long time. So be patient. If it is going to take you two months to eat an apple every day, how long is it going to take your child with autism to automatically make the right behavior choice?

Follow Your Plan; Sometimes Things Get Worse Before They Get Better

You may have discovered that when you start a new behavior plan, the behaviors get worse before they get better. This is often true when you decide to ignore a problem behavior, called an "extinction burst." But it can also happen when any new plan is started. You may see a temporary increase in the problem behavior, and it appears that what you're doing is not working, or even making things worse. But be patient and don't give up! Your plan may take time and multiple trials to work.

On the other hand, if you know you have consistently followed the plan and, after several weeks, your data show that your child's behavior has not improved, then you may need to make changes. A professional can also help you work through the following questions.

Refining Your Plan

There are a multitude of reasons why some plans work and others don't. Remember that each person with autism is different so what works for one might not work with another. Here are some ideas to consider.

1. Is the problem specific enough? Remember to be as specific as you can.

2. Do the problem and the plan fit the Rule of Five?

3. Have you identified the right reason for the problem? Remember not to make assumptions but to gather facts.

4. Have you identified an appropriate and reasonable replacement behavior, skill, or new rule? Is it specific enough for your child to understand? Are the steps clear? Are smaller steps needed?

5. Are you practicing the new plan with your child in advance of when he needs it?

6. Have you assessed and modified the environment? Remember that changing the antecedents often prevents the problem in the first place.

7. Are you using visual supports to communicate the expected behavior and new plan? Are they clear and specific enough?

8. Is your verbal communication clear?

9. Is more predictability or preparation needed?

10. Are you using praise and other words of encouragement regularly?

11. Are you using powerful reinforcers at the appropriate time intervals?

12. Are you using punishment or other negative consequences when your child has not mastered the skill(s) you are asking of him? Remember that the use of negative consequences is only permissible when the child has mastered the skills in multiple environments.

13. Is it time to consider medication support?

⚙ Rule: Don't give up. Get help!

If you are struggling and your plan isn't working, find help. There are numerous types of specialists, and choosing the best person(s) for you and your child requires careful consideration. Look for a specialist who is certified in his or her profession, is experienced with autism and challenging behaviors, has a good reputation in your community, is willing to collaborate with others, and is committed to evidence-based interventions. Be sure to request references.

Your insurance company's patient service representative, as well as most primary care providers, teachers and mental health professionals will be able to assist you or refer you to someone who can. If they cannot, contact your local autism society for the names of experts and resources in your area. Also, consult the Helpful Information at the end of this book.

In the meantime, focus on your child's strengths, what he or she can do well. Support positive behaviors with praise and encouragement, and remember that behavior change WILL happen. Be sure to take time for yourself and other family members. They need you too and can help lighten your load. Please keep your sense of humor.

Final Thoughts – From Surviving to Thriving

Hopefully, you have moved from "Yes, but . . . ." (all of the arguments why you and your child cannot change) to "Yes, and . . ." (all of the strategies that you and your child need to try). Autism is a lifelong condition, not life long imprisonment; your child CAN learn! With your efforts and the help of others around you, problems can be managed, skills can be learned and you and your child can thrive. Remember the Rule of Five and make the plan fit your child; there is no "one size fits all." Finding your way will take some time, but equipped with the rules and tools in this book your journey will be smoother. Remember that the impact of your efforts will be life changing – for your child and for your family.

BEHAVIOR

Problem Description

1. Problem Behavior: _____

2. Rule of Five: Will the problem matter in five weeks, five months, or five years? Yes/No

   Why or why not? _____

3. When is the problem most and least likely to occur?

   Most: _____

   Least: _____

4. Where is the problem most and least likely to occur?

   Most: _____

   Least: _____

5. With whom is the problem most and least likely to occur?

   Most: _____

   Least: _____

6. The significance of the problem is ☐Mild ☐Moderate ☐Severe ☐Extreme

7. The reasons for the problem include: _____

   _____

8. The possible antecedents for this problem are: ☐ Environment ☐Sensory ☐Communication ☐Physical/Biological ☐Required Skills ☐Required Knowledge

   Detailed Description: _____

   _____

Interventions

1. Antecedent modifications might include: _____

   _____

2. What exactly do I want the child to do instead of the problem behavior? _____

   _____

3. The replacement behavior(s), new rule(s), new skill(s), or new routine(s) to be practiced and reinforced are:

   ☐ _____

   ☐ _____

   ☐ _____

4. The type of reward program is:

    ☐ Primary rewards

    The menu of rewards will include: (include the amount of reward)

    ○ _____

    ○ _____

    ○ _____

    ☐ Secondary rewards are: _____, which will be exchanged for:

    ○ _____

    ○ _____

    ○ _____

5. The schedule of reinforcement is: _____

6. The communication plan includes:

    ☐ Visual schedule

    ☐ Visual supports/tool(s)

    ○ _____

    ○ _____

    ○ _____

    ☐ Verbal strategies

    ○ _____

    ○ _____

    ○ _____

7. The consequences for the problem behavior will be:

☐ Redirection	☐ Natural consequences
☐ Logical consequence	☐ Withholding reinforcement
☐ Loss program	☐ Timeout
☐ None at this time	☐ Other

8. Medication supports are:

    ☐ None

    ☐ _____

9. Ongoing data collection and monitoring of the plan will occur on the:

☐ Daily Behavior Log	☐ Problem Behavior Record
☐ Weekly Behavior Log	☐ Behavior Information Tool
☐ Behavior Significance Scale	☐ Sleep Chart
☐ Medication Effect Checklist	☐ Other

Teaching New Skills and Routines

1. One new/unexpected/stressful situation for my child is: _____

    _____

    The preparation plan will include:

    ☐ Getting Ready Checklist

    ☐ Priming for "What If?"

2. One "Now and Forever" skill/task/routine to teach my child is: _____

    _____

    All of the following are prepared and ready to use to teach:

    ☐ The task analysis (write out the steps of the task).

    ☐ Decision: backward/forward chain?

    ☐ Reward system:

        ☐ Primary rewards

           The menu of rewards will include: (include the amount of reward)

           ○ _____

           ○ _____

           ○ _____

        ☐ Secondary rewards are: _____, which will be exchanged for:

           ○ _____

           ○ _____

           ○ _____

    ☐ Visual tool(s)

        ○ _____

        ○ _____

    ☐ Materials: _____

    ☐ Setting: place: _____

    ☐ Context: link between skill and need to teach it: _____

    ☐ Time: when _____

    ☐ People who will teach: _____

    ☐ Directions: clear steps in visual format: _____

    ☐ Method to monitor success and problems. _____

3. A detailed master schedule for daily routines is written and agreed upon. Yes/No

4. The 1-3 social skills to focus teaching will be:

☐ Ask for help	☐ Ask a question on the topic
☐ Be a good sport	☐ Give and receive compliments
☐ Greet (beginner/intermediate)	☐ Join in
☐ Offer encouragement	☐ Share
☐ Wait	☐ Work in a group
☐ Other _____	☐ Other _____

5. The teaching plan will include:

☐ Social Skills Daily Practice Log

☐ Skills Steps

☐ Reward system:

   ☐ Primary rewards

   The menu of rewards will include: (include the amount of reward)

   ○ _____

   ○ _____

   ○ _____

   ☐ Secondary rewards are: _____, which will be exchanged for:

   ○ _____

   ○ _____

   ○ _____

☐ Visual tool(s)

   ○ _____

   ○ _____

   ○ _____

☐ Materials: _____

☐ Settings: _____

☐ Context: link between skill and need to teach it: _____

☐ Time: when _____

☐ People who will teach: _____

☐ Practice activities will include:

   ○ _____

   ○ _____

   ○ _____

References and Further Reading

Lally, P., van Jaarsveld, C.H.M., Potts, H.W.W., & Wardle, J. (2010). How are habits formed: Modeling habit formation in the real world. *European Journal of Social Psychology, 40,* 998-1009.

Complete List of the Rules

Chapter 1: Behavior and Autism

1. Behavior communicates.

2. Most children learn behaviors from their environment.

3. No two children with autism are alike.

4. Children with autism share a unique set of behavior characteristics, yet there are no "typical" behavior challenges.

5. Interventions that work for one child with autism may not work for another.

6. Children with autism like predictability and routine.

7. The Rule of Five: Predict five weeks, five months, and five years into the future.

Chapter 2: The Problem

8. Be as specific as you can when describing the problem.

Chapter 3: Is the Behavior Significant?

9. Frequency, duration, intensity, setting, and persistence help determine the significance of a problem.

Chapter 4: Determining Why: Reasons for the Behavior

10. Don't make assumptions: Gather facts.

11. Step back, listen, and watch.

12. Behavior has a purpose.

Chapter 5: The Power of Antecedents

13. Changing the antecedents – what happens before the behavior – often prevents the problem in the first place.

14. Teach skills instead of punishing behavior.

15. Decide exactly what you want the child to do, not just what you don't want the child to do.

Chapter 6: Effective Communication

16. Visual communication helps to communicate more effectively.

17. Visual tools help retain information.

18. Visual tools reduce the number of verbal directives needed.

19. Visual tools highlight what is important.

20. Visual tools improve organization.

21. Rules for giving directions, commands, and demands

    a. Be clear.

    b. Get the child's attention.

    c. Be positive.

    d. Make the last word count and eliminate contractions.

    e. Slow things down. Reduce your language.

    f. Tell the child what you want him to do (instead of what you don't want him to do).

    g. Prompt BEFORE the unacceptable behavior happens.

    h. Use "real" choices.

    i. Use specific, not general, time references.

    j. Add extra information.

    k. Don't give a directive if you don't have time to follow through.

    l. Praise and reward compliance.

    m. Practice.

Chapter 7: Teaching New Rules

22. Sometimes the expected behavior is not as obvious to the child as it is to you.

23. Everyone involved must know the new rule(s).

Chapter 8: Using Praise and Primary Rewards

24. Behavior that is followed by a reward is more likely to occur again.

25. Praise builds confidence.

26. Give attention for positive behavior.

27. Use more encouragement than criticism.

28. Be specific with your praise.

29. Praise effort, not just success.

30. Use small amounts of the reward.

31. Choose a powerful reward for a new program.

32. To reinforce high-frequency new behaviors, use small amounts of the reward.

33. Reward attempts and approximations.

34. Limit access to the reward.

Chapter 9: Using Secondary Rewards

35. Choose specific behaviors to reward with tokens, points, or other secondary rewards.

Chapter 10: Building Flexibility

36. Multiple unanticipated events can create a crisis for the child with autism.

37. Reducing the total number of unexpected events in a day helps to reduce cumulative stress.

38. Getting ready for new experiences is the key to success.

39. Flexibility = More than one right way.

Chapter 11: Changing Routines and Fixations

40. If you don't make up the rule, the child may do it for you.

41. What is seemingly obvious to others is not obvious to some children with autism.

Chapter 12: "Now and Forever"

42. Start teaching early.

43. Teach the right way from the start.

44. Begin with small and specific tasks.

45. Set the child up to succeed by preparing in advance.

46. Use rewards.

47. Use task analysis and behavior chains.

48. Teach one step at a time.

49. Be consistent and follow through every day.

50. Keep track of progress.

51. Determine reasons for any problems.

52. Create "now and forever" routines.

Chapters 13 and 14: Teaching Social Skills Parts I and II

53. Social skills require direct teaching, just like other skills.

54. Teaching is everyone's job, including you.

55. The context determines what skills are needed.

56. Fundamental skills are integrated parts of other skills.

57. Social skill deficits are one reason for challenging behavior.

58. Identify specific skills for focused teaching.

59. Emphasize the positive, not the negative.

60. Arrange for practice activities at home.

61. Arrange for practice activities in the community.

62. Teach "now and forever" social rules.

Chapter 15: Using Consequences

63. Negative consequences, when used alone, do not permanently change behavior in most children with autism.

64. Sometimes consequences reinforce misbehavior.

65. Selecting consequences should be the last step of the plan, not the first.

66. Children with autism who learn and use skills in one environment may not automatically use them in another.

67. Negative consequences are only permissible when a child has mastered a skill or behavior in multiple environments.

68. Timeout works best when a child has mastered the skill or task being asked *and* he wants to be with family members and friends.

69. Timeout should never be the only intervention.

70. When timeout is reinforcing, the child is likely to engage in the misbehavior again.

Chapter 16: Medication support

71. Medication is a supportive treatment in autism, not a primary treatment.

72. Gather as much information about the medication as you can.

73. Change one intervention approach at a time.

74. Response to medications is often different for children with autism than for typically developing children.

Chapter 17: The Final Chapter: Putting It All Together

75. Behavior change takes time.

76. Don't give up. Get help!

Relating the Tools to the National Autism Center's (NAC) Standards Report

The four-tier rating system developed by the NAC to describe the level of effectiveness of autism treatments and the descriptions includes:

1. **Established.** Sufficient evidence is available to confidently determine that a treatment produces beneficial treatment effects for individuals on the autism spectrum. That is, these treatments are established as effective.

2. **Emerging.** Although one or more studies suggest that a treatment produces beneficial treatment effects for individuals with ASD, additional high quality studies must consistently show this outcome before we can draw firm conclusions about treatment effectiveness.

3. **Unestablished.** There is little or no evidence to allow us to draw firm conclusions about treatment effectiveness with individuals with ASD. Additional research may show the treatment to be effective, ineffective, or harmful.

4. **Ineffective/Harmful.** Sufficient evidence is available to determine that a treatment is ineffective or harmful for individuals on the autism spectrum.

From http://www.nationalautismcenter.org/pdf/NAC%20Standards%20Report.pdf

Using this rating system the NAC identified 11 Established Treatments, 22 Emerging Treatments, 5 Unestablished Treatments, and 0 Ineffective/Harmful Treatments. The relationship(s) between each rule in the book and its main corresponding NAC treatment category is described in the table below (occasionally there is more than one main NAC treatment category).

The definitions of the key NAC treatment categories include the following

Established Treatments

Antecedent Package – These interventions involve the modification of situational events that typically precede the occurrence of a target behavior. These alterations are made to increase the likelihood of success or reduce the likelihood of problems occurring. Treatments falling into this category reflect research representing the fields of applied behavior analysis (ABA), behavioral psychology, and positive behavior supports.

Behavioral Package – These interventions are designed to reduce problem behavior and teach functional alternative behaviors or skills through the application of basic principles of behavior change. Treatments falling into this category reflect research representing the fields of applied behavior analysis, behavioral psychology, and positive behavior supports.

Modeling – These interventions rely on an adult or peer providing a demonstration of the target behavior that should result in an imitation of the target behavior by the individual with ASD. Modeling can include simple and complex behaviors. This intervention is often combined with other strategies such as prompting and reinforcement. Examples include live modeling and video modeling.

Schedules – These interventions involve the presentation of a task list that communicates a series of activities or steps required to complete a specific activity. Schedules are often supplemented by other interventions such as reinforcement. Schedules can take several forms including written words, pictures or photographs, or work stations.

Self-management – These interventions involve promoting independence by teaching individuals with ASD to regulate their behavior by recording the occurrence/non- occurrence of the target behavior, and securing reinforcement for doing so. Initial skills development may involve other strategies and may include the task of setting one's own goals. In addition, reinforcement is a component of this intervention with the individual with ASD independently seeking and/or delivering reinforcers. Examples include the use of checklists (using checks, smiley/frowning faces), wrist counters, visual prompts, and tokens.

Emerging Treatments

Exposure – These interventions require that the individual with ASD increasingly face anxiety-provoking situations while preventing the use of maladaptive strategies used in the past under these conditions.

Social Skills Package – These interventions seek to build social interaction skills in children with ASD by targeting basic responses (e.g., eye contact, name response) to complex social skills (e.g., how to initiate or maintain a conversation)

From http://www.nationalautismcenter.org/pdf/NAC%20Standards%20Report.pdf

Tools		NAC Treatment Categories	Established	Emerging	How the Tool Relates to NAC Standards
\multicolumn{6}{c}{**Chapter 2: The Problem**}					
1.	**Daily behavior log**	Behavioral Package	X		Provides a structured method to gather data about behavior
\multicolumn{6}{c}{**Chapter 3: Is the Behavior Significant?**}					
2.	**Weekly behavior log**	Behavioral Package	X		Provides a structured method to gather data about behavior
3.	**Behavior significance scale**	Behavioral Package	X		Provides a structured method to gather data about behavior significance
\multicolumn{6}{c}{**Chapter 4: Determining Why: Reasons for the Behavior**}					
4.	**Problem behavior record**	Behavioral Package	X		Provides a structured method to gather data about reasons for problem behavior
5.	**Behavior information tool**	Behavioral Package	X		Provides a structured method to gather data about behavior
6.	**Sleep chart**	Behavioral Package	X		Provides a structured method to gather data about sleep behavior
\multicolumn{6}{c}{**Chapter 5: The Power of Antecedents**}					
7.	**Antecedent checklist**	Antecedent Package	X		Provides a list of common variables affecting a problem
\multicolumn{6}{c}{**Chapter 6: Effective Communication**}					
8.	**Visual schedule/visual supports**	Schedules	X		Provides a visual list to check the events of the day
9.	**Giving directions**	Behavioral Package	X		Utilizes cueing and prompting to teach behavior
		Antecedent Package	X		Utilizes specific format to increase likelihood of successful task completion
\multicolumn{6}{c}{**Chapter 7: Teaching New Rules**}					
10.	**Wrong way/right way**	Behavioral Package	X		Utilizes cueing and prompting to teach replacement behaviors
		Antecedent Package	X		Utilizes visual support to increase likelihood of positive behavior
11.	**Red words and green words**	Behavioral Package	X		Utilizes cueing and prompting to teach replacement behaviors
		Antecedent Package	X		Utilizes visual support to increase likelihood of positive behavior
12.	**Out & about**	Behavioral Package			Utilizes cueing and prompting to teach appropriate behavior in public
		Antecedent Package	X		
			X		Utilizes visual support to increase likelihood of positive behavior
\multicolumn{6}{c}{**Chapter 8: Using Praise and Primary Rewards**}					
13.	**Reward survey**	Behavioral Package	X		Detects potential positive reinforcers
14.	**Activity survey**	Behavioral Package	X		Detects potential positive reinforcers
15.	**Visual support tool**	Schedules	X		Provides a visual reminder of the accepted behavior and the reinforcement

Chapter 9: Using Secondary Rewards					
16.	**Secondary rewards (i.e., tokens)**	Behavioral Package	X		Creates motivation to engage in positive behavior
17.	**Point system**	Behavioral Package	X		Creates motivation to engage in positive behavior through use of a token economy
18.	**Reward card**	Behavioral Package	X		Creates motivation to engage in positive behavior and practice new skills
19.	**Contract**	Behavioral Package	X		Creates motivation to engage in positive behavior
20.	**Allowance**	Behavioral Package	X		Creates motivation to engage in positive behavior and learn new skills
Chapter 10: Building Flexibility					
21.	**Getting ready**	Antecedent Package	X		Priming for new activities and unfamiliar circumstances
		Schedule	X		Provides a concrete list of steps to prepare for a new activity or unfamiliar event
22.	**Think out loud**	Modeling	X		Demonstrates target behavior
23.	**Model positive self-talk**	Modeling	X		Demonstrates target behavior
24.	**Visual supports**	Antecedent Package	X		Provides a visual demonstration of alternative choices to promote problem solving
25.	**"What if"**	Antecedent Package	X	X	Priming or preparation for new activities and unfamiliar circumstances
		Exposure Package			Uses pre-teaching to reduce anxiety when faced with stressful situation
Chapter 11: Changing Routines and Fixations					
26.	**Determine a new rule**	Antecedent Package	X		Modifies the event to reduce likelihood of problems
27.	**Change the routine**	Antecedent Package	X		Provides choice, priming and environmental modification
		Behavioral Package	X		Promotes reinforcement for the new behavior routine
Chapter 12: Now and Forever					
28.	**Self-help and independent skills checklist**	Behavioral Package	X		Provides a list of skills needed for independent functioning and records the amount of help needed to perform them
29.	**Preparing in advance**	Antecedent Package	X		Provides a structured method to set up the environment to increase likelihood of successful teaching
30.	**Task analysis**	Behavioral Package	X		Teaches new skills through the identification of specific steps in each task
31.	**Behavior chains**	Behavioral Package	X		Teaches new skills through the step-by-step teaching of each part in a behavior chain
32.	**Master schedule for routines**	Antecedent Package	X		A structured method to set up the environment to increase likelihood of reduced problems
		Schedule	X		Provides a visual list of the day's routines
Chapter 13: Teaching Social Skills Part I					
33.	**Super skills**	Social Skills Package		X	Builds social interaction by targeting specific skills to teach
		Behavioral Package	X		Teaches replacement behaviors
34.	**Social skills daily practice log**	Self-Management	X		Identify individual skills that encourage interaction

Chapter 14: Teaching Social Skills Part II					
35.	**Skills steps**	Social Skills Package		X	Identify behaviors that comprise social skills
		Antecedent Package	X		Provide cues and prompts to engage with others in multiple settings
		Schedules	X		Provide a visual list of steps to each skill
36.	**Rewards**	Behavioral Package	X		Create motivation to engage in social interaction
37.	**Modeling**	Modeling	X		Uses adult and peer/sibling demonstration
38.	**Practice activities**	Social Skills Package		X	Promote social initiation, social response and getting along with others in a positive practice environment
Chapter 15: Using Consequences					
39.	**Consequence strategies**	Behavioral Package	X		Used to respond to behaviors in ways that do not maintain the problem behavior
40.	**Timeout procedure**	Behavioral Package	X		Procedure to remove attention and reinforcement for a problem behavior
Chapter 16: Medication Supports					
41.	**Medication effect checklist**	NAC report is not applicable*			Helps to identify and evaluate medication treatment effects and monitor any adverse effects
Chapter 17: The Final Chapter: Putting It All Together					
42.	**Master Action Plan (MAP)**	Behavioral Package	X		Provides a structured method to describe the problem, interventions and data collection tools

* The NAC committee did not address medication supports.

Helpful Information

Practical Books and Websites for Parents & Caregivers

General

Johnston-Tyler, J. (2007). *The mom's guide to asperger syndrome and related disorders.* Shawnee Mission, KS: AAPC Publishing.

Koegel, L. K., & LaZebnik, C. (2004). *Overcoming autism: Finding the answers, strategies and hope that can transform a child's life.* New York, NY: Penguin Books.

Emotion Regulation

Baker, J. (2008). *No more meltdowns.* Arlington, TX: Future Horizons.

Dacey, J. S., & Fiore, L. B. (2000). *Your anxious child: How parents and teachers can relieve anxiety in children.* San Francisco, CA: Jossey-Bass Publishers.

Dunn Buron, K. (2007). *A 5 could make me lose control.* Shawnee Mission, KS: AAPC Publishing.

Gardner, L., & Jaffe, A. (2006). *How to control and react to the size of your emotions – An interactive workbook for parents, professionals, and children.* Shawnee Mission, KS: AAPC Publishing.

Lineham, H. J., Wignall, A., & Rapee, R. M. (2008). *Helping your anxious child children's workbook* (2nd ed.). Sydney, AU: Centre for Emotional Health, Macquarie University.

Manasco, H. (2006). *The way to A: Empowering children with autism spectrum and other neurological disorders to monitor and replace aggression and tantrum behavior.* Shawnee Mission, KS: AAPC Publishing.

Myles, B. S., & Southwick, J. (2005). *Asperger syndrome and difficult moments: Practical solutions for tantrums, rage and meltdowns* (2nd ed.). Shawnee Mission, KS: AAPC Publishing.

Rapee, R. M., Wignall, A., Spence, S. H., Cobham, V., & Lyneham, H. (2008). *Helping your anxious child: A step-by-step-guide for parents* (2nd ed.). Oakland, CA: New Harbinger Publications, Inc.

General Behavior Strategies

Cardon, T. (2008). *Top ten tips: A survival guide for families with children on the autism spectrum.* Shawnee Mission, KS: AAPC Publishing.

Fouse, B., & Wheeler, M. (1997). *A treasure chest of behavioral strategies for individuals with autism.* Arlington, TX: Future Horizons.

Mayaya, K., & Owens, P. (2013). *Successful problem-solving for high-functioning students with autism spectrum disorder.* Shawnee Mission, KS: AAPC Publishing.

Sakai, K. (2005). *Finding our way: Practical solutions for creating a supportive home and community for the Asperger syndrome family.* Shawnee Mission, KS: AAPC Publishing.

Independence and Self-Help Skills

Baker, B. L., & Brightman, A. J. (1989). *Steps to independence: A skills training guide for parents and teachers of children with special needs* (2nd ed.). Baltimore, MD: Paul H. Brookes.

Coucouvanis, J. (2008). *The potty journey: Guide to toilet training children with special needs, including autism and related challenges.* Shawnee Mission, KS: AAPC Publishing.

Hudson, J., & Bixler Coffin, A. (2007). *Out and about: Preparing children with autism spectrum disorders to participate in their communities.* Shawnee Mission, KS: AAPC Publishing.

Orth, T. (2006). *Visual recipes – A cookbook for non-readers.* Shawnee Mission, KS: AAPC Publishing.

Medications

Tsai, L. Y. (2001). *Taking the mystery out of medications in autism/asperger syndromes: A guide for parents and non-medical professionals.* Arlington, TX: Future Horizons.

Social Skills Assessment: Tools to Identify Specific Skills to Target for Intervention

Social Skills Checklist: In Quill, K. (2000). *Do-watch-listen-say: Social and communication intervention for children with autism.* Baltimore, MD: Brookes Publishing.

Autism Social Skills Profile: In Bellini, S. (2006). *Building social relationships: A systematic approach to teaching social interaction skills to children and adolescents with autism spectrum disorders and other social difficulties.* Shawnee Mission, KS: AAPC Publishing.

Profile of Social Difficulty: In Coucouvanis, J. (2005). *Super skills: A social skills group program for children with Asperger syndrome, high-functioning autism and related challenges.* Shawnee Mission, KS: AAPC Publishing.

Social Skill Menu: In Baker, J. (2005). *Preparing for life: The complete guide for transitioning to adulthood for those with autism and Asperger's Syndrome.* Arlington, TX: Future Horizons.

Social Skills Training at Home and in the Community

Baker, J. (2003). *The social skills picture book.* Arlington, TX: Future Horizons.

Baker, J. (2003). *Social skills training for children and adolescents with Asperger Syndrome and social-communication problems.* Shawnee Mission, KS: AAPC Publishing.

Baker, J. (2005). *Preparing for life: The complete guide for transitioning to adulthood for those with autism and asperger's syndrome.* Arlington, TX: Future Horizons.

Baker, J. (2006). *Social skills picture book for high school and beyond.* Arlington, TX: Future Horizons.

Bareket, R. (2006). *Playing it right! Social skills activities for parents and teachers of young children with autism spectrum disorders, including Asperger Syndrome and autism.* Shawnee Mission, KS: AAPC Publishing.

Buron, K. D. (2007). *A 5 is against the law! Social boundaries – Straight up! An honest guide for teens and young adults.* Shawnee Mission, KS: AAPC Publishing.

Coucouvanis, J. (2005). *Super skills: A social skills group program for children with Asperger Syndrome, high-functioning autism and related challenges.* Shawnee Mission, KS: AAPC Publishing.

Diamond, S. (2011). *Social rules for kids-the top 100 social rules kids need to succeed.* Shawnee Mission, KS: AAPC Publishing.

Gray, C. (2001). *My social stories book.* Philadelphia, PA: Jessica Kingsley Publishing.

Gregson, B. (1982). *The incredible indoor games book.* Carthage, Ill: Fearon Teacher Aids.

Gregson, B. (1984). *The outrageous outdoor games book.* Torrance CA: Fearon Teacher Aids.

Madrigal, S., & Winner, M. G. (2008). *Superflex, a superhero social thinking curriculum.* San Jose, CA: Think Social Publishing, Inc.

Myles, B. S., & Hudson, J. (2007). *Starting points: The basics of understanding and supporting children and youth with Asperger syndrome.* Shawnee Mission, KS: AAPC Publishing.

Myles, B., Schelvan, R. L., & Trautman, M. (2013). *The hidden curriculum for understanding unstated rules in social situations for adolescents and young adults* (2nd ed.). Shawnee Mission, KS: AAPC Publishing.

Quill, K. (2000). *Do-watch-listen-say: Social and communication intervention for children with autism.* Baltimore, MD: Brookes Publishing.

Weiss, M., & Harris, S. L. (2001). *Reaching out, joining in: Teaching social skills to young children with autism.* Bethesda, MD: Woodbine House.

Winner, M. G. (2007). *Thinking about you, thinking about me. Second edition.* San Jose, CA: Think Social Publishing, Inc.

Visual Supports

Bernard-Opitz, V., & Häußler, A. (2011). *Visual support for children with autism spectrum disorders: Materials for visual learners.* Shawnee Mission, KS: AAPC Publishing.

Hodgdon, L. A. (1995). *Visual strategies for improving communication, Volume 1: Practical supports for school and home.* Troy, MI: QuirkRoberts Publishing.

Hodgdon, L. A. (1999). *Solving behavior problems in autism: Improving communication with visual strategies.* Troy, MI: QuirkRoberts Publishing.

Publishers That Specialize in Autism and Related Disabilities

AAPC Publishing
11209 Strang Line Road
P.O. Box 23173
Lenexa, KS 66215
Phone: 877-277-8254
Website: www.aapcpublishing.net

Brookes Publishing Co.
P.O. Box 10624
Baltimore, MD 21285-0624
Phone: 800-638-3775
Website: www.brookespublishing.com

Future Horizons, Inc.
721 West Abram Street
Arlington, TX 76013

Phone: 800-489-0727
Website: www.fhautism.com

Jessica Kingsley Publishers
400 Market Street, Suite 400
Philadelphia, PA 19106
Phone: 866-416-1078
Website: www.jkp.com

Woodbine Publishing House
6510 Bells Mill Road
Bethesda, MD 20817
Phone: 800-843-7323
Website: www.woodbinehouse.com

Distributors of Visual Communication and Educational Materials

Attainment Company
504 Commerce parkway
P.O. Box 930160
Verona, WI 53593-0160
Phone: 800-327-4269
Website: http://www.attainmentcompany.com
Products: Pictured materials, software for daily living, community access and skill building, assistive technology

Different Roads to Learning
37 East 18th St., 10th Floor
New York, NY 10003
Phone: 800-853-1057
Website: http://www.difflearn.com
Products: Educational materials, communication boards, schedules, individual picture cards, token boards, timers, assistive technology

Do2Learn
3204 Churchill Road
Raleigh, NC 27607
Phone: 919-755-1809
Website: http://www.dotolearn.com/
Products: Free pages with social skills and behavioral regulation activities and guidance, learning songs and games, communication cards, academic material, and transition guides for employment and life skills. In addition, View2do, JobTIPS, FACELAND

Don Johnston Company
26799 W. Commerce Drive
Volvo, IL 60073
Phone: 800-999-4660
Website: http://www.donjohnston.com
Products: Educational software and FACELAND, b-Calm, Improv, Co:Writer, Picture This

EnableMart
School Health Corporation Customer Service
865 Muirfield Drive
Hanover Park, IL 60133
Phone: 888-640-1999
Website: http://www.enablemart.com
Products: Communication software

Intellitools, Inc.
1720 Corporate Circle
Petaluma, CA 94954
Phone: (800) 899-6687
Website: http://www.intellitools.com
Products: Educational software – IntelliKeys, Stages, Overlay Maker, ReadyMade Story Kits, Math Pad

Jessica Kinsley Publishers
400 Market Street, Suite 400
Philadelphia, PA 19106
Phone: 866-416-1078
Website: http://www.jkp.com
Products: ISPEEK at Home; ISPEEK at School

Kid Access
6526 Darlington Road
Pittsburgh, PA 15217
Phone: 412-521-8552
Website: http://www.kidaccess.com
Products: Eye-cons (a collection of drawings on CD-ROM or customized printout)

Mayer-Johnson Company
P.O. Box 1579
Solana Beach, CA 92075-7579
Phone: 800-588-4548
Website: http://www.mayer-johnson.com
Products: Boardmaker; Picture Communication Symbols (PCS) and PCS books. Software – Visual Essentials, Places You Go, Things You Do; toolkit of clip art; video sign language dictionary

Pyramid Educational Products Inc.
13 Garfield Way
Newark, DE 19713
Phone: 888-732-7462
Website: http://www.pecs.com
Products: Pics for PECS, Schedule boards, communication books, visual supports

Silver Lining Multimedia, Inc.
P.O. Box 544
Peterborough, NY 03458
Phone: 888-777-0876
Website: http://www.silverliningmm.com
Products: Picture This; Places You Go, Things You Do; Functional Living Skills; School Routines and Rules, Visual Foods; and Visual Essentials

Suncastle Technology
3475 Bridge Road, Suite 8-438
Suffolk, VA 23435
Phone: 877-306-6968
Website: www.suncastletech.com
Products: Software – Picture It (adds symbols to text); PixWriter

Tech4Learning
10981 San Diego Mission Road, Suite 120
San Diego, CA 92108
Phone: 877 834-5453
Website: http://pics.tech4learning.com/
Products: Free image library for education

Time-Timer
7707 Camargo Road
Cincinnati, OH 45243
Phone: 877-771-TIME (8463)
Website: http://www.timetimer.com/contact.
php#sthash.1r410LwQ.dpuf
Products: Timers in various format that visually show time, time lapse, etc.

Useful Websites

Autism Society: www.autism-society.org/ works to increase public awareness about autism and the day-to-day issues faced by people with autism and their families. They provide information and education, support research and advocate for programs and services for the autism population. The Autism Society has state and local chapters. Call toll-free 1-800-328-8476.

Autism Speaks www.autismspeaks.org/ is dedicated to funding global biomedical research into the causes, prevention, treatments, and cure for autism and to raising public awareness about autism and its effects on individuals, families, and society.

Centers for Disease Control: www.cdc.gov/ncbddd/autism/provides information for families, people with ASD, health care providers, educators and policy makers, including facts, screening and diagnosis, treatment, data and statistics, research, links, etc.

Family Drug Guide: http://www.unboundmedicine.com/products/family_drug_guide/ is an easy-to-use application that provides information to help you discuss medications, ask the right questions, and make the best decisions with your healthcare provider.

First Signs: www.firstsigns.org/is dedicated to educating parents and professionals about autism and related disorders. The First Signs website provides information on a range of issues: from monitoring development, to concerns about a child, from the screening and referral process, to sharing concerns.

Interactive Autism Network: www.iancommunity.org/ was established at Kennedy Krieger Institute and is funded by a grant from Autism Speaks. IAN's goal is to facilitate research that will lead to advancements in understanding and treating autism spectrum disorders.

Medline Plus: http://www.nlm.nih.gov/medlineplus/druginformation.html/ is the National Institutes of Health's Web site for reliable, up-to-date information on drugs and supplements. It is produced by the National Library of Medicine.

National Autism Center: www.nationalautismcenter.org/is dedicated to serving children and adolescents with Autism Spectrum Disorders by providing reliable information, promoting best practices, and offering comprehensive resources for families, practitioners, and communities.

National Institute of Mental Health: http://www.nimh.nih.gov/health/publications/a-parents-guide-to-autism-spectrum-disorder/index.shtml/ presents an overview of autism for parents with links to research opportunities.

National Dissemination Center for Children with Disabilities: http://nichcy.org/ is a central source of information on disabilities, including early intervention, special education and related services, IEPs, family issues, disability organizations, professional associations, education rights, transition to adult life, and more. They provide personal answers to your questions, fact sheets, state resource sheets, parent guides, reading lists, and referrals to other organizations. Materials are also available in Spanish. Call toll-free 1-800-695-0285.

Quackwatch: www.quackwatch.com/ is a nonprofit corporation whose purpose is to combat health-related frauds, myths, fads, and fallacies. Information on quackery, questionable therapies.

Treatment and Education of Autism and related Communication-handicapped Children (TEACCH): www.teacch.com/ is an evidence-based service, training, and research program for individuals of all ages and skill levels with autism spectrum disorder.

Zero to Three: www.zerotothree.org/is a national non-profit organization providing resources on the first three years of life, with a mission to strengthen and support families, practitioners and communities to promote the healthy development of babies and toddlers.

100 Useful Sites, Networks, and Resources for Parents of Autistic Children: www.mastersinhealthcare.com/blog/2009/100-useful-sites-networks-and-resources-for-parents-of-autistic-children/

National Reports

National Standards: http://www.nationalautismcenter.org/pdf/NAC%20Standards%20Report.pdf

The Interagency Autism Coordinating Committee Strategic Plan for Autism Spectrum Disorder Research – 2012 Update, U.S. Department of Health and Human Services: http://iacc.hhs.gov/strategic-plan/2012/index.shtml

Index

A

Antecedent
 Checklist, 54, 63
 Definition, 42
 Power of, 53-61
 Preparing, 150

B

Behavior
 Information tool, 50
  Chain, 152-154
 Daily Behavior Log, 22
  Definition, 5-6
 Function, 45-46
 Intent, 197-198
 Problem Behavior Record, 49
  Replacement, 81-84, 102, 199, 202
  Reasons for, 47
  Significance Scale, 35
  Statements, 15-17
  Weekly Behavior Log, 36

C

Co-occurring conditions, 210

Communication
 Verbal, 73-77
 Visual, 65-72, 85

Consequence(s), 27, 43, 53, 102, 110
  Strategies, 199

F

Flexibility, 119-130
Functional analysis, 59

H

Hidden curriculum, 81, 174

M

Master Action Plan, 231-234
Medication
  As additional treatment, 209
  Effect (antecedent checklist), 63
  Effect Checklist, 219

P

Preparation/priming, 111, 121-122, 124

R

Reward/reinforcement
 Amount of, 103
  Menu, 98
 Obsessive interests as, 98
  Schedule, 104
  Surveys, 99-101
  Types, 93-94, 112
Routine
 Changing, 133-138
 Creating, 67, 68, 109, 110, 127, 130
 Disruption in, 56, 85, 120
 Need for, 8, 57
Rule of Five, 9, 10, 28, 33, 58, 59, 124, 135, 141

S

Schedules
 Changing, 129, 130
 Daily, 68, 69, 151
  First and Then, 69
 Mini, 72, 138
 Master Schedule for Routines, 157
Self-Help & Independent Skills Checklist, 145-148
Skills
 Components, 152, 167
 Deficits, 57, 64, 141, 163
 Task analysis, 152
Sleep
 Chart, 44, 45, 51

Difficulties with, 44, 55
Medications for, 217
Social skills
Daily Practice Log, 169
Context, 63, 88, 150, 165
Getting along with others, 166-167
Social initiation, 166-167
Social response, 166-167
Stress and anxiety
Coping with, 126
Medications for, 217
Model, 121
Parent testimonial, 72, 131
Reason for behavior, 47, 129, 170
Structure
Need for, 133, 156

T

Timeout
Log, 207
Procedure, 202
Rules, 201

V

Visual communication/support, 65-67, 85, 102,
111, 127, 128

Related Books From AAPC

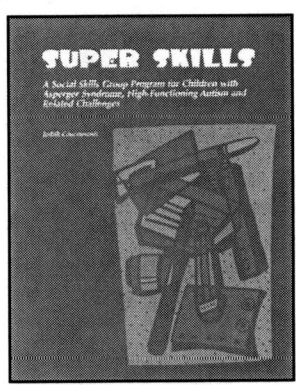

Super Skills

A Social Skills Group Program for Children With Asperger Syndrome, High-Functioning Autism and Related Challenges

by Judith Coucouvanis, MA, APRN, BC; foreword by Brenda Smith Myles, PhD

This series of social skills activities are designed to help elementary-aged students with autism spectrum and other social-cognitive deficits succeed in the social realm. Each lesson is highly structured and organized, making it easy for teachers and other group leaders to implement successfully. A series of practical checklists and other instruments provide a solid foundation for assessing students' social skills levels and subsequent program planning.

ISBN 9781931282673 | Code 9937 | Price: $39.95

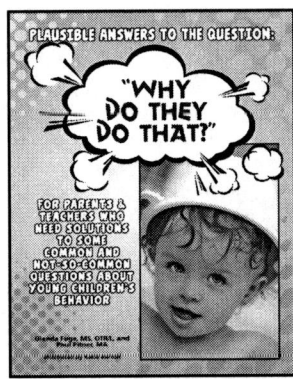

Plausible Answers to the Question: "Why Do They Do That?"

For parents & teachers who need solutions to some common and not-so-common questions about young children's behavior

by Glenda Fuge, MS, OTR/L, and Paul Pitner, MA

This is a hands-on reference for parents, other caregivers, and teachers, that takes a unique approach to children's behaviors that often dismay and puzzle adults. Using a practical and reader-friendly format, the book presents each behavior, such as crying, on a two-page spread within clear and easy-to-read sections such as Question, Plausible Answers (does it stem from social, sensory, communication issues), Basic Training (suggestions for what to do), and Over and Above (further ideas, who to consult in serious cases, etc.). Applicable to children five years old and younger.

ISBN 9781937473860 | Code 9114 | Price: $22.95

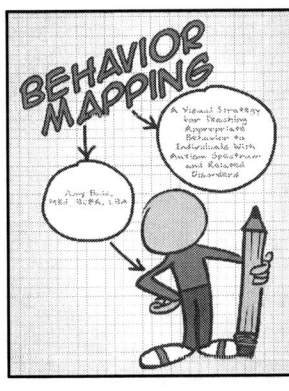

Behavior Mapping

A Visual Strategy for Teaching Appropriate Behavior to Individuals With Autism Spectrum and Related Disorders

by Amy Buie, MEd, BCBA, LBA

Playing to the visual strengths of students with autism spectrum and related disorders and their need for structure and consistency, Behavior Mapping helps children make good choices with regard to their behavior by visually showing them available options and the consequences for each action they choose at any given time. Due to its visual nature, this strategy, whether paired with written and/or oral directions, is effective for a range of students, regardless of age and ability level. Built upon evidence-based practices, their are three major types of Behavior Maps – Consequence Maps, Language Maps, and Problem-Solving Maps, each serving a different purpose aligned with common areas of difficulty for students with social-cognitive challenges.

ISBN 9781937473822 | Code 9107 | Price: $19.95

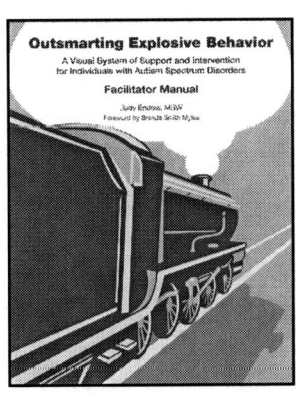

Outsmarting Explosive Behavior

A Visual System of Support and Intervention for Individuals With Autism Spectrum Disorders

by Judy Endow, MSW; foreword by Brenda Smith Myles, PhD

Outsmarting Explosive Behavior is a visual program, laid out as a fold-out poster that can be personalized for each user. Four train cars represent stages of explosive behavior: Starting Out, Picking up Steam, Point of No Return and Explosion. This program, which also includes a how-to handbook and student workbook, makes it easy to help individuals identify their current state and take steps to decrease the chances of a meltdown.

ISBN 9781934575444 | Code 9035 | Price: $34.95

To order, please visit www.aapcpublishing.net

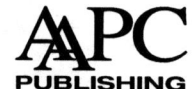

PUBLISHING

P.O. Box 23173
Shawnee Mission, Kansas 66283-0173
www.aapcpublishing.net

CPSIA information can be obtained at www.ICGtesting.com
Printed in the USA
LVOW09s0157200914

404851LV00002B/3/P

9 781937 473853